"I know one thing for sure, Anthony Moses is real, his message is authentic, and his book will transform your life. Failing to plan is planning to fail but this journal is the solution to life's challenges, whether spiritual, emotional, physical or whatever. I owe a big thank you to Anthony for his dedication and excellence at teaching health in all of its aspects. You will too."

Joel Kahn, MD, FACC
Founder, Kahn Center for Cardiac Longevity
Clinical Professor or Medicine, Wayne State University School of Medicine

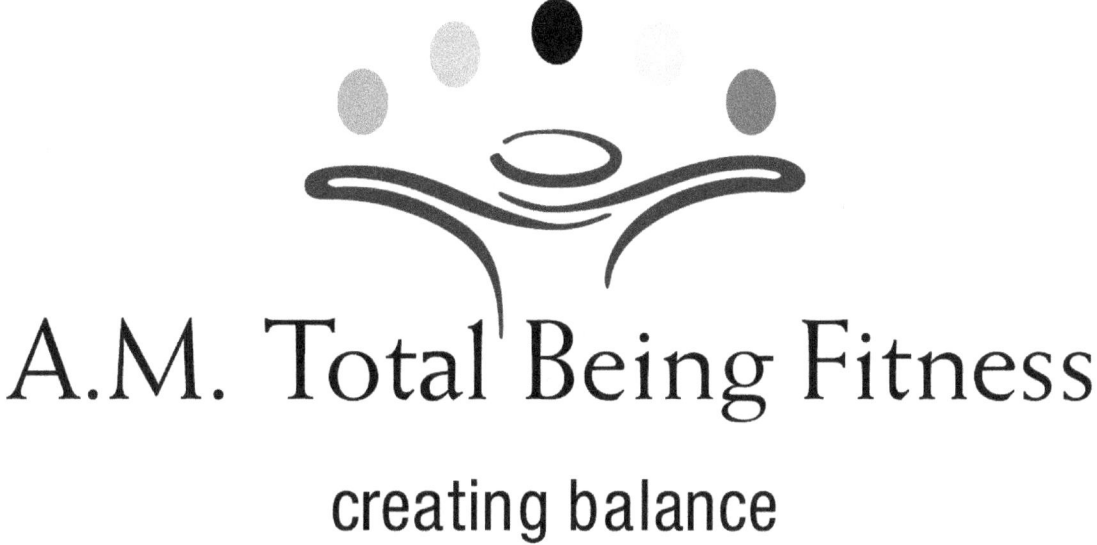

Copyrighted Material
A.M. Total Being Fitness: creating balance
Copyright © 2018 Anthony Moses
All Rights Reserved

No part of this publication may be reproduced, stored in a retrieval system
or transmitted, in any form or by any means — electronic, mechanical, photocopying,
recording, or otherwise — without prior written permission from the publisher,
except for the inclusion of brief quotations in a review.

For information about this title or to order other books
and/or electronic media, contact the publisher:

Atkins & Greenspan Publishing
18530 Mack Avenue, Suite 166
Grosse Pointe Farms, MI 48236
www.atkinsgreenspan.com

ISBNs
978-1-945875-34-3 (Paperback)
978-1-945875-35-9 (eBook)

Printed in the United States of America

© 2008, 2018 by Anthony Moses
© Cover Design Van-garde Imagery, Inc.
© Back Cover credit

Photographs used with permission.

The Five Elements of the Total Being

Spiritual
Meditation, prayer, gratitude, patience. These help us to become more understanding of what we feel within ourselves and those around us.

Emotional
The mind often travels to the past and sometimes to the future where we revisit past or anticipate future emotions. Being aware of and understanding how this makes us feel will help us create more balance within ourselves.

Physical
Our body is our vehicle in this life. We maintain our cars so they run efficiently and for as long as we can drive them; why not show our bodies the same care and respect so they run as efficiently.

Social
Our social surroundings are also our support system. We want to surround ourselves with positive, caring, and loving people. Remember to communicate with your spouse, your friends, your family and pay attention to how you feel before and after social interactions.

Intellectual
To keep our sharpest mental focus, we must manage our daily lives, plan our activities week ahead in order to keep our personal and work lives organized, and create routines that will help keep balance throughout the day, the week, the month.

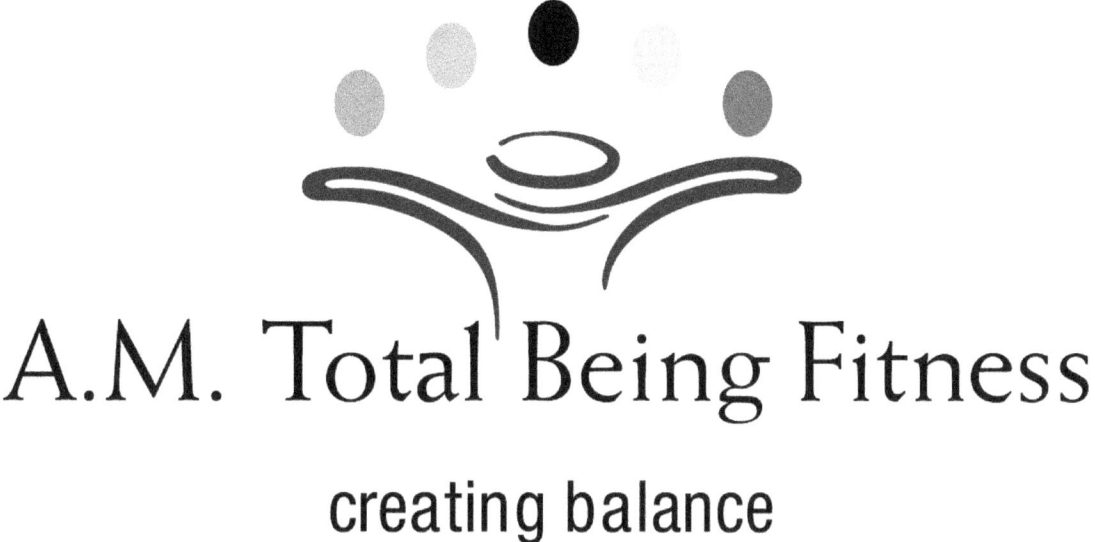

A.M. Total Being Fitness
creating balance

A Journal

Anthony Moses

About Anthony's Total Being Program: Is It Right for Me?

Anthony's Total Being Program is not for those who are looking for a workout routine or some formula for change. In fact, Anthony's approach is based on the premise that to change one's body, one must change one's thinking, one's emotions, and one's spirit. The message is basic – but it is not simple – and it is the truth that all of us know deep down inside.

Everyone knows that diet and exercise must go together. Likewise, working out and dieting while continuing to put unhealthy experiences, beliefs, words, and people in our lives is still an incomplete and ineffective strategy.

Watching what we put in our mouths but not watching what else we put in our lives is a recipe for disaster.

Anthony's style of personal training is passionate and spiritual. His insights and his philosophy of change incorporate not just biological and physiological facts about fitness but also:

- Evolutionary theories about animals' instincts and natural trends towards survival;

- Creationism and an awareness of that non-physical part of us that makes us human;

- Developmental psychology perspectives that explain the connection between our emotions and our beliefs;

- Sociological explanations about the impact of environment on a person's thoughts, feelings, and behaviors;

- Historical and political observations about the causes and effects of cultural unity and disharmony in the world;

- Concepts from Eastern medicine applied to the interrelatedness of the mind and the body.

Anthony's views are backed by his own success and the transformation of many of his clients. In his own experience, his body has changed more than he ever imagined possible. Paradoxically, he does not *see* the change as much as he *feels* that everything clicks for him and life is easier.

Anthony's thinking and training may seem unconventional (i.e., *Don't count reps!*) and his metaphors are more like Zen koans than instructions (*The spirit is the direction; the mind is the driver; and the body is just the vehicle*), but his Total Being idea has something to offer everyone.

About Anthony

As owner and founder of A.M. Total Being Fitness, I've drawn on my own life experiences and 15 years of work in the fitness industry to develop a program that is truly unique.

At the age of 11, I was diagnosed with Crohn's disease and given two years to live by my doctors. At the age of 16, I was determined to take myself off all medications and heal myself through faith, exercise, diet, attitude, and healthy relationships. I have been medication-free for nearly 30 years, enjoying a healthy and rewarding lifestyle.

My team and I strive to help our members safely and effectively lose weight, get strong, make changes in their lives and feel great. We have developed a warm, motivating & enthusiastic style and approach to fitness that has helped many people weed through all the hype and learn what really works.

I have presented, as a motivational speaker, for Oakwood Hospital, DMC Childrens' Hospital, Detroit Lions, Detroit City Council and many local businesses in Dearborn, Michigan.

Certifications

- American Council in Exercise (A.C.E.), - Certification for Personal Training
- Wellness Coac
- AFFA Certified Trainer
- Certified Nutrition Specialist
- Core Strength Certification
- Shiatsu Stretching Certification
- Longevity Wellness Specialist
- CPR Certified

Accomplishments -

- Featured in the *Detroit News, Detroit Free Press*, ABC Channel 7 with Carolyn Clifford
- National Gym Association Overall Champion 2006

- 5th Place Muscle Mania International
- Top 5 in the National Physique Committee's Team Universe for 2002, 2003, 2004
- 1st Place Detroit Muscle Mania 2003
- Mr. Michigan 2001 Body Building Overall Champion
- 1st Place Mr. Ohio 2001 Body Building Champion
- Iron Man 2001 Body Building Overall Champion

The Importance of Journaling

Our routines get us from one day to the next. Yet, how many of us take a moment to *feel* where we are when we wake up in the morning or before we go to sleep at night? Journaling is an important activity that helps us stay in the present moment; journaling can get us from one day to the next; and journaling can help us have the clarity to understand what we are feeling and why we are feeling it.

Have you ever had a morning when everything seems to go wrong? By the end of the night you may be extremely stressed out and tense, but you cannot understand why, even if you had a productive day at work?

If you are journaling, you will be able to reflect and recognize the emotions that you experienced throughout your day. This understanding will allow you to relax and rest at the end of the night.

Journaling also helps you set goals and track them to determine whether you have reached them or not.

Journaling allows for personal growth and helps you explore who you really are so you can be in touch with your inner self.

If you've never journaled before, don't worry. You can start with the basics: just the facts. You can write down what time you got up, how you felt, what you ate, and so on throughout the day.

You are the best to judge your best time of day to journal. Whether you write at bedtime or throughout the day is your choice. Do what feels right, and you're more likely to repeat it, and make it a habit.

Don't be concerned about "getting it right." It's more important to start!

creating balance

At the End of this Program, You will Have Some Tools

When we eliminate outside things, it brings us closer to inside of self.

Spiritual: Praying, repenting, meditating, listening to the voice that is the inner you, accepting and loving who you are, fasting from food, hobby's and sex.

Emotional: Paying attention to how you feel when you are around others and you feel in the moment of expressing and staying in touch with your emotions. When we express our emotions, we let

Physical: Paying attention to what we put in our bodies and noticing how it makes us feel physically, which effects our body flow (to brain), circulation (to muscles), oxygen (chemical balance). When we eat right, we feel better.

In the old days and the in the rain forest, people are happy just surviving, breathing fresh air, walking, hunting their food. They are getting all kinds of exercise being surrounded by others like themselves; they are not affected socially by life. If we eat right, think right, act right surround ourselves with people like us, we then become whole and that is true happiness.

Total Being Test

Part 1

This is a *Total Being* test. It will help you look at what you consider to be most important in your life. Please rate the following elements on a scale of 1-5, with 1 being the most important to you and 5 being the least important. *Note: there are no wrong answers!*

... Physical (Appearance and how you look/feel) E

... Emotional (How you feel) X

... Intellectual (How you think and learn) Y

... Spiritual (How you see and perceive things on a higher level of understanding) H

... Social (People, work, functions, friends, etc.) Z

creating balance

Total Being Test

Part 2

Please rate the following elements on a scale of 1-5, with 1 being the most important to you and 5 being the least important. *Note: there are no wrong answers!*

... Family (Spouse, children, parents, siblings, etc.) X

... Finances (Money, possessions, etc.) Y

... Friends (associates, intimates, etc.) Z (might need some clarification)

... Faith (Beliefs, determination, resilience, etc.) H

... Health (Eating habits, activity level, rejuvenation, etc.) E

Answer Key: Total Being Test

Part 1

Compare how you ranked the Five Elements of Total Being in your life with the answer key analysis below:

Spiritual – What your ranking indicates:

1. If you ranked Spiritual as #1, you are on the right path. You have determination, willpower, disposition, and the faith to succeed.

2. If you ranked *Spiritual* as #2, you may be lacking determination, willpower, disposition, and faith.

3. If you ranked *Spiritual* as #3, you are probably beginning to go down the wrong path.

4. If you ranked *Spiritual* as #4, most likely you have had to endure some hardships in the past.

5. If you ranked *Spiritual* as #5, you are on the wrong path. You need to make a change now or you will continue to experience a destructive lifestyle

Physical – What your ranking indicates:

1. If you ranked *Physical* as #1, you put too much emphasis on your outside appearance.

2. If you ranked *Physical* as #2, you put your body above the way feel on the inside.

3. If you ranked *Physical* as #3, your physical outlook is in line with what you want.

4. If you ranked *Physical* as #4, you tend to put material things above your health.

5. If you ranked *Physical* as #5, you put yourself last and/or have low self-esteem.

Social – What your ranking indicates:

1. If you ranked *Social* as #1, you tend to care too much about what other people think.

2. If you ranked *Social* as #2, you think other people come before you and how you feel.

3. If you ranked *Social* as #3, you allow others' behaviors, opinions, and actions to strongly affect your own behavior.

4   If you ranked *Social* as #4, you are in control of your social behavior.

5   If you ranked *Social* as #5, people around you affect how you feel.

Intellectual – What your ranking indicates:

1   If you ranked *Intellectual* as #1, you tend to put too much emphasis on money and things.

2   If you ranked *Intellectual* as #2, your priorities are not in order.

3   If you ranked *Intellectual* as #3, you are thinking too much.

4   If you ranked *Intellectual* as #4, you doubt your decision-making skills quite often.

5   If you ranked *Intellectual* as #5, you have your thinking in perspective and are on track.

Emotional – What your ranking indicates:

1   If you ranked *Emotional* as #1, You put your emotions in front of what is real. You are overly sensitive.

2   If you ranked *Emotional* as #2, you are completely in tune with your emotions.

3   If you ranked *Emotional* as #3, you put your emotions last and hid from your feelings.

4   If you ranked *Emotional* as #4, you are not in touch with your emotions.

5   If you ranked *Emotional* as #5, you are not in touch with yourself at all. You often experience sad, empty, or "dead" feelings.

Diet for Spiritual Health

1. Be grateful for the life that has been given to you.

2. Repent and ask for forgiveness for the things you have done wrong.

3. Be aware of your surroundings, including the people in your life.

4. Fast/abstain from TV, music, food – the things you enjoy. This will enable you to experience the void and appreciate them more.

5. Pray and give thanks.

6. Do onto others as you would have them do to you.

7. Forgive and love.

8. Try to understand that everything happens because of an action.

9. Ask yourself, "Why?" not "Why me?" Recognize that everything happens for a reason. Learn and grow from it.

10. Have faith, hope, determination, and willpower.

11. Surround yourself by people who have the same values and beliefs that you have.

creating balance

Diet for Emotional Health

1. Try to understand your history – where your ancestors came from.

2. Try to understand what they had to go through and how it affected them.

3. Take a good look at your parents. Learn from them and their experiences.

4. Know that you reflect your parents because you are part of them.

5. Accept who you are. Love the things that you cannot change about yourself – try to understand those things.

6. Realize that you are always growing — and so are others around you.

7. Allow yourself to express how you feel. Stay true to yourself and others.

8. Always reflect on your day and plan for your tomorrow.

9. Remember that a thought can trigger and emotion. You can change your thoughts to positive ones to change your emotions.

10. As an emotional outlet, do things you loved to do as a child.

11. Remember that too much focus on any of the following is a negative way to cope with problems or voids in your life, including:

    l. Alcohol
    m. Blaming others
    n. Clothes/external appearance
    o. Drugs – street and prescription
    p. Entertainment
    q. Excuses
    r. Food
    s. Greed
    t. Lies
    u. Lust
    v. Money
    w. Toys/Worldly possessions
    x. Work

Diet for Physical Health

1. Move your body every day. Live a more active lifestyle. Climb the stairs instead of taking the elevator.

2. Remember that not exercising your body each day is like not brushing your teeth.

3. Do cardiovascular activities for at least 30 minutes three times a week. Gradually increase your activity time and frequency.

4. Lift weights at least two times a week. Gradually increase the amount and frequency you lift over time.

5. Take part in leisure activities that are physical – tennis, golf, basketball, biking, kickboxing, or dancing.

6. Make exercise a priority by fitting it into your daily schedule and keep the appointment!

7. Do not use physical appearance in negative ways, such as for advancement.

8. Take care of your physical body, but do not obsess over it. Remember that the body is just the wrapping of your true gift – your spirit.

9. Remember that a healthy body can enhance your spiritual self by allowing your inside to shine through.

Diet for Social Health

1. Be aware of your associates' and friends' beliefs. They can affect you.

2. If people make you feel bad or uncomfortable continually, do not hang around them.

3. Just because everyone is doing it, doesn't mean it is the right thing to do.

4. When you open yourself up emotionally, you will be socially affected.

5. Be selective and only try to be around people who have a similar direction as you in life.

6. Remember that friction occurs when people do not have similar life directions.

Diet for Intellectual Health

1. Use your knowledge and skills in a positive way, but not to simply benefit yourself.

2. Try to use your capabilities to benefit others, especially those in need.

3. Stay open minded. When you think you know everything, you know nothing.

4. Remember that your way is not the only way. Oftentimes, two heads are better than one. You can build off others' ideas.

5. Before you lay down at night and get out of bed in the morning, recognize that how you feel is real.

6. Use your intellectual ability to understand why you feel a certain way.

7. Come up with positive ways to deal with negative emotions.

8. Use your intellectual ability to plan ahead. Plan time for exercise. Plan time to prepare healthy meals and snacks. Prepare your meals for a week at a time, for example, on Sunday.

9. Do not skip breakfast. You cannot work well when your body is low on energy/food.

How to Journal

Here's an example of how to use a journal. This single page tells the story of Pam's day.

Pam's Journal
Monday.

- Woke up 15 minutes late – hit the snooze button too many times. My morning started in a blur. I got in the shower, dressed for work, and rushed out the door.

- At work, I was called into a meeting as soon as I got to my desk. I had a minute to grab a quick cup of coffee. Such a busy morning, I didn't realize I hadn't eaten till my stomach growled in the meeting.

- Worked through lunch. Didn't get around to eating until after 1:30 p.m. I went to the cafeteria and grabbed a sandwich, a bag of chips, and a soda, which I ate at my desk while working on my To-Do pile.

- Tried to push through till the end of the day, but grabbed a snack from the vending machine (I was tired and hungry) about 30 minutes before I left for the day.

- At home, I realized the fridge is empty, and I need to go grocery shopping. I looked at the clock, and thought it was too late (I didn't have the energy), so I just called and ordered a pizza.

- After pizza, I drank glass of wine to unwind.

- Flipped channels on the TV. A little later, I went to bed.

As you can see, Pam recorded the most basic details. If she wanted, she could look back over her day and see where she might make changes if she so desired.

creating balance

How to Journal for Self Assessment

Using the Five Elements:
Spiritual • Emotional • Physical • Social • Intellectual

Each day take a few minutes to reflect on the five elements of your life. Jot down positive and negative influences and/or experiences of the day. Think about what YOU can do differently to reduce or change the negative and promote more positive. Then put your plan into ACTION!

Spiritual

What this encompasses: Meditation, prayer, gratitude, patience.

Benefits: These help us to become more understanding of what we feel within ourselves and those around us.

Your spiritual self is often described as *a belief in a higher being or one's faith*. You can strengthen your spirituality through practicing your religion, prayer, or meditation. If you are open minded, your spirituality can even be enhanced through life's experiences. For example, when you share in the miracle and joy of the birth of a baby or grieve and reflect on the life of someone who dies, you can experience spirutal growth.

Emotional

What this encompasses: The mind travels to the past and sometimes to the future.

Benefits: Being aware of where our mind travels and understanding how it makes us feel will help us create more balance within ourselves.

Your emotions are *how and what you feel*. Expressing laughter or anger allows us to grow just as when we feel pain and cry. Our emotional component is strongly influenced by the four other realms.

Physical

What this encompasses: Our body is our vehicle in this life.

Benefits: We maintain our cars so they run efficiently and for as long as we can drive them; why not show our bodies the same care and respect so they run as efficiently.

Your physical capability is *what your body is able to do*. When you train, you overload your cardiovascular and respiratory systems. This increase your ability to take in more oxygen which is necessary for your body to function. When we lift weight, we overload our muscles and increase our strength. Alas: No pain, no gain!

Social

What this encompasses: Our social surroundings are also our support system.

Benefits: We want to surround ourselves with positive, caring, and loving people. Remember to communicate with your spouse, your friends, your family and pay attention to how you feel before and after social interactions.

Your social self includes your environment, including *what surrounds you and the people you interact with*. For example, rain and sunshine enable life on earth to growth. A plan will not grow if it does not get enough water and sunlight. You, too, will not grow if you are surrounded by things that prevent your growth.

When you surrounded yourself by gloom and doom and negative people, you can start to feel negative. However, you can turn negative experiences into positive ones. For example, if someone takes advantage of you, just learn from the experience and your mistakes. This enables you to grow and become wiser.

Intellectual

What this encompasses: To keep our sharpest mental focus.

Benefits: We must manage our daily lives, plan our activities week ahead in order to keep our personal and work lives organized, and create routes that will help keep balance throughout the day, the week, the month.

Your intellectual self is *what you know*. The more you read, the more knowledge you gain. If you are able to apply what you learn and not just *know* it, you are even further ahead.

Here is a guide for using the Five Elements to delve deeply into your day. Let's use Pam's Journal as our example:

Spiritual: Did you pray/meditate today? Have you asked for forgiveness for yourself and forgiven others? Have you been grateful and thankful for your blessings? Have you been grateful for the life that has been given to you and do you understand that everything happens for a reason?

Let's take Pam's Journal entry and delve more deeply:

Positive

I am grateful for my job.

Negative

I did not have time to pray or meditate today because I was rushed all day long.

Plan of Action

Tomorrow I plan to wake up early enough to make time for myself in the morning and meditate so I can have a clear mind before I get started.

Emotional: Did you take a moment to yourself in the morning to pay attention to how you felt, before you started your day? Did you express your emotions instead of suppressing them? Did you acknowledge and allow yourself to feel and experience a range of emotions appropriately, without overreacting? Did you understand the emotions that you felt and not allow them to take you to your past?

Positive

I told my boss that I had a rough morning and she was very understanding. That relieved some of my stress when I first got in.

Negative

My day was such a blur; I can't really remember all of my encounters.

Plan of Action

I will make sure I step away from my work and encounters with co-workers throughout my day to pay attention to how I am feeling.

Physical: Did you take care of yourself today? Did you eat six small meals? Did you exercise? Did you smoke? Did you drink alcohol? Did you eat fast food?

Positive

I was able to take a shower and get ready for work.

Negative

I did not have time to workout or eat breakfast. I also did not get a chance to go grocery shopping and I ending up skipping many meals and eating very unhealthy foods. I had one glass of wine.

Plan of Action

Tomorrow, I will get up early enough to prepare my breakfast, lunch, and snacks and will make time to go grocery shopping. I will stop by the gym after work and do my cardio.

Social: Who were you around socially? How did it make you feel? Did you limit your exposure to negative surroundings and understand what you felt? Did you give in to negative influences?

Positive

My boss was very understanding when I told her that I woke up late and was rushing to work. That relieved some of my worry about my productivity and attentiveness at work today.

Negative

Some of the people in the office were talking about the economy. Their opinions were negative, and that irritated me.

Plan of Action

I will spend more time focusing on my work and will limit my time around negative surroundings. If I am in a negative surrounding I can't leave right away, I will try to put out some optimism.

Intellectual: Did you plan your day out by writing it down? Did you plan ahead to exercise? Did you prepare your meals and healthy snacks? Did you skip breakfast because you were rushing to work? Did you choose an unhealthy snack because you didn't prepare? Don't forget to take time to yourself, before you go to sleep, to recognize what you are feeling!

Positive

I am journaling before I go to sleep, so I can wake up with clarity tomorrow.

Negative

Today was bad. I did not plan and ended up with a very poor diet, skipped meals, didn't exercise, and had a lot of unnecessary stress.

Plan of Action

I will get up early enough to write my day out tomorrow morning.

Your Starting Point

If you don't know where you are going, how long will it take you to get there?

Name: _____

Starting Date: _____

Starting Weight: _____

Goal Weight: _____

Starting Body Fat %: _____

Goal Body Fat %: _____

Goals for your Five Elements of Life:

Spiritual:

_____

_____

_____

Emotional:

_____

_____

_____

A.M. Total Being Fitness

Physical:

_____

_____

_____

Social:

_____

_____

_____

Intellectual:

_____

_____

_____

creating balance

The Road to Success

Things you will need:

- Food Scale
- Plastic Containers
- Small Cooler
- Workout Music
- Good quality running shoes
- CD Player/MP3 Player
- Realistic Goals
- Time commitment for workouts and meal planning

Things you need to do – Eating Tips:

1. Have your body fat checked first before starting any nutritional program so you can eat the right amount of each nutrient for your body type and personal goals.

2. Read labels.

3. Plan meals for the week or at least 2-3 days in advance.

4. Eat breakfast.

5. Eat 6-8 times a day.

6. Eat fruit or power bars for snacks.

7. Eat 30 – 50 grams of fiber each day by gradually increasing the amount you eat so your body can adjust to avoid gas, cramping, and diarrhea.

8. Drink 8 – 16 (8-ounce) glasses of water a day, at least 64 ounces.

9. Try not to consume more than 4 ounces of protein per meal.

10. Do not skip meals! More calories are burned when you eat at regular intervals. Just do not overeat! When you do not eat, your metabolism (how fast energy is burned) slows down.

Foods to stay away from:

- *All fast food*
- Deep-fried food
- Refined flours and starches
- Sugar and sweets
- Sugar-laden beverages

Food suggestions for meals:

- Breakfast – eggs or oatmeal
- Snacks – fruit, nuts, yogurt, kefir cheese, cottage cheese
- Lunch/Dinner – Chicken, fish, tuna, rice or potato

Nutrient content of common foods per serving:

Food	g CHO (Carbohydrates)	g PRO (Protein)	Fat
Eggs (1)	0	6	5
Chicken (4 oz. skinless)	0	28	5
Fish (3 oz. lean)	0	21	2
Turkey (4 oz.)	0	28	2-4
Brown Rice (2/3 cup)	33	1	3
Fruit (1 piece or 1/2 cup)	15	0	0
Vegetables (1/2 cup)	5-10	2	0
Oatmeal (1/2 cup)	27	5	3
Whole Wheat Pasta (2/3 cup)	40	7	1
Potatoes (1 medium)	33	3	1
Corn/Peas (1/2 cup)	15	3	0
Salad (1 cup)	5	0	0
Rice Cake with 1 tsp Peanut Butter and Honey	20	2	4

Facts to Remember:

1. When you train at 80% of your maximum heart rate, you burn about 80% of sugar and 20% fat.

2. The more good fat you eat the more stored fat you burn. When you do cardio, the fat around your waist is the fat that is used for energy first.

3. Water is the most important nutrient used by your body. You could go several days without food and still survive, but go 3-4 days without water and you will die! So, remember to drink up!

4. Nutrients help chemical reactions occur in your body. Your brain is 80% water and your body is about 65%. We are water (substance = life), muscle (protein), bones (minerals), and cell membranes and padding around organs (fat). Do not eliminate any nutrients from your diet! They all play important roles.

The key to success:

- Assess the five elements of your life daily.
- Plan and act on ways to improve as needed.
- Follow the diets for the 5 elements of life.
- Record your food intake.
- Keep an open mind.
- Stay true to yourself.
- Entrust yourself to your spirit and you will succeed!

creating balance

Food Exchange List

https://www.nhlbi.nih.gov/health/educational/lose_wt/eat/fd_exch.htm

You can use this list to give yourself more choices.

Very Lean Protein

Fruits/ Lean Protein

Medium Fat Proteins

Starches

Fats

Note:
1-gram of cho = 4 cal

1-gram of pro = 4 cal

1-gram of fat = 9 cal

Breakfast/Snack

Fat-Free and Very Low-fat Milk - One serving

1 cup milk, fat-free or 1% fat

¾ cup yogurt, plain nonfat or lowfat

1 cup yogurt, artificially sweetened

Fruits - One serving

1 small apple, banana, orange, nectarine

1 medium fresh peach

1 kiwi

½ grapefruit

½ mango

1 cup fresh berries (strawberries, raspberries or blueberries)

1 cup fresh melon cubes

⅛ honeydew melon

4 ounces unsweetened juice

4 teaspoons jelly or jam

1 each whole egg (medium) **

1 ounce mozzarella cheese

¼ cup ricotta cheese

4 ounces tofu (note this is a heart healthy choice)

** choose these very infrequently

Lunch/Dinner

Vegetables - One serving

1/2 cup cooked vegetables (carrots, broccoli, zucchini, cabbage, etc.)

1 cup raw vegetables or salad greens

1/2 cup Vegetable juice

If you're hungry, eat more fresh or steamed vegetables

Very Lean Protein - One serving

4 ounces turkey breast or chicken breast, skin removed

4 ounces fish fillet (flounder, sole, scrod, cod, etc.)

4 ounces canned tuna in water

4 ounces shellfish (clams, lobster, scallop, shrimp)

3/4 cup cottage cheese, nonfat or low fat

4 each egg whites

1/4 cup egg substitute

1 ounce fat-free cheese

1/2 cup beans - cooked (black beans, kidney, chick peas or lentils)

4 ounces chicken- dark meat, skin removed

4 ounces turkey- dark meat, skin removed

4 ounces salmon, swordfish, herring

4 ounces lean beef (flank steak, London broil, tenderloin, roast beef)*

4 ounces veal, roast or lean chop*

4 ounces lamb, roast or lean chop*

Dinner/Lunch

Lean Protein – One serving

1 ounce low-fat cheese (3 grams or less of fat per ounce)

1 ounce low-fat luncheon meats (with 3 grams or less of fat per ounce)

1/4 cup 4.5% fat cottage cheese

2 medium sardines

* Limit to 1-2 times per week

Starches – One serving at a time

1 slice bread (whole wheat, rye)

2 slice reduced calorie or "lite" Bread

1/4 (1 ounce) bagel (varies)

1/2 English muffin

3/4 cup cold cereal

2/3 cup rice, brown cooked

2/3 cup barley or couscous - cooked

1/2 cup pasta - cooked

2/3 cup legumes (dried beans, peas or lentils) - cooked

1/2 cup bulger - cooked

1/2 cup corn, sweet potato or green peas

3 ounces baked sweet or white potato

3/4 ounce pretzels

3 cups popcorn, hot air popped or microwave (80% light)

Fats - One serving at a time

1 teaspoon Oil (vegetable, corn, canola, olive, etc.)

1 teaspoon Butter

1 teaspoon Stick margarine

1 teaspoon Mayonnaise

1 Tablespoon reduced fat margarine or mayonnaise

1 Tablespoon Salad dressing

1 Tablespoon Cream cheese

2 Tablespoons Lite cream cheese

1/8 Avocado

8 large olives (black)

10 large olives (stuffed green)

A.M. Total Being Fitness

Meal Journal

Day 1   Date: _____

Quote of the Day: *Being "fit" is more than what we see on the outside!*

Meal 1   Time _____   Protein _____

_____   Complex CHO _____

_____   Simple CHO _____

_____   Fat _____

Water _____   Sodium _____

Meal 2   Time _____   Protein _____

_____   Complex CHO _____

_____   Simple CHO _____

_____   Fat _____

Water _____   Sodium _____

Meal 3   Time _____   Protein _____

_____   Complex CHO _____

_____   Simple CHO _____

_____   Fat _____

Water _____   Sodium _____

creating balance

Meal 4   Time _____   Protein _____

_____   Complex CHO _____

_____   Simple CHO _____

_____   Fat _____

Water _____   Sodium _____

Meal 5   Time _____   Protein _____

_____   Complex CHO _____

_____   Simple CHO _____

_____   Fat _____

Water _____   Sodium _____

Meal 6   Time _____   Protein _____

_____   Complex CHO _____

_____   Simple CHO _____

_____   Fat _____

Water _____   Sodium _____

Total Daily Caloric Intake:

Calories _____

Water _____

_____ gms Carb

_____ gms Protein

_____ gms Fat

Exercise Journal

Cardio

Type of Cardio: _____

Duration: _____

Intensity: _____

Calories Burned: _____

Type of Cardio: _____

Duration: _____

Intensity: _____

Calories Burned: _____

Weight Training

Type of Exercise: _____

Reps: _____

Sets: _____

Amount of Weight: _____

Type of Exercise: _____

Reps: _____

Sets: _____

Amount of Weight: _____

Type of Exercise: _____

Reps: _____

Sets: _____

Amount of Weight: _____

Type of Exercise: _____

Reps: _____

Sets: _____

Amount of Weight: _____

Type of Exercise: _____

Reps: _____

Sets: _____

Amount of Weight: _____

creating balance

Self-Assessment Journal

Reflect on the 5 elements of your life. Jot down positive and negative influences and/or experiences of the day. Think about what YOU can do differently to reduce or change the negative and promote more positive. Then put your plan into ACTION!

Spiritual: Did you pray/meditate today? Have you asked for forgiveness for yourself and forgiven others? Have you been grateful and thankful for your blessings? Have you been grateful for the life that has been given to you and do you understand that everything happens for a reason?

Positive

_____

_____

_____

Negative

_____

_____

_____

Plan of Action

_____

_____

_____

Emotional: Did you take a moment to yourself in the morning to pay attention to how you felt, before you started your day? Did you express your emotions instead of suppressing them? Did you acknowledge and allow yourself to feel and experience a range of emotions appropriately, without overreacting? Did you understand the emotions that you felt and not allow them to take you to your past?

Positive

_____
_____
_____

Negative

_____
_____
_____

Plan of Action

_____
_____
_____

Physical: Did you take care of yourself today? Did you eat six small meals? Did you exercise? Did you smoke? Did you drink alcohol? Did you eat fast food?

Positive

Negative

Plan of Action

Social: Who were you around socially? How did it make you feel? Did you limit your exposure to negative surroundings and understand what you felt? Did you give in to negative influences?

Positive

_____
_____
_____

Negative

_____
_____
_____

Plan of Action

_____
_____
_____

Intellectual: Did you plan your day out by writing it down? Did you plan ahead to exercise? Did you prepare your meals and healthy snacks? Did you skip breakfast because you were rushing to work? Did you choose an unhealthy snack because you didn't prepare? Don't forget

Positive

Negative

Plan of Action

What is a Workout?

A workout is 25% perspiration
and 75% Determination.
Stated another way, a workout is one part physical exertion
And three parts self-discipline.
Doing it is easy once you get started.

A workout makes you better today
than you were yesterday.
It strengthens the body, relaxes the mind
and toughens the spirit.
When you workout regularly,
your problems diminish and your self confidence grows.

A workout is a personal triumph
over laziness and procrastination.
It is a badge of a WINNER and the mark of an organized,
goal-oriented person
who has taken charge of his or her DESTINY.

A workout is a wise use of time
and an investment in excellence.
It is a way of preparing for life's challenges
and proving to yourself
that you have what it takes to do whatever is necessary.

A workout is a key that helps unlock the door to opportunity and SUCCESS.
Hidden within each one of us is an extraordinary force.
Physical and mental fitness are the triggers
that release that force.

A workout is a form of rebirth.
When you finish a good workout,
you don't simply feel better…

YOU FEEL BETTER ABOUT YOURSELF.

creating balance

Meal Journal

Day 2   Date: _____

Quote of the Day: *Before you lose the weight, you must lose what lies underneath it. This includes the hate, resentment, anger, pride, etc. If you do not lose these underlying emotions, you will experience those same emotions later on and end up the same way you were before.*

Meal 1   Time _____

_____

_____

_____

Water _____

Protein _____

Complex CHO _____

Simple CHO _____

Fat _____

Sodium _____

Meal 2   Time _____

_____

_____

_____

Water _____

Protein _____

Complex CHO _____

Simple CHO _____

Fat _____

Sodium _____

Meal 3   Time _____

_____

_____

_____

Water _____

Protein _____

Complex CHO _____

Simple CHO _____

Fat _____

Sodium _____

Meal 4   Time _____

_____

_____

_____

Water _____

Protein _____

Complex CHO _____

Simple CHO _____

Fat _____

Sodium _____

Meal 5   Time _____

_____

_____

_____

Water _____

Protein _____

Complex CHO _____

Simple CHO _____

Fat _____

Sodium _____

Meal 6   Time _____

_____

_____

_____

Water _____

Protein _____

Complex CHO _____

Simple CHO _____

Fat _____

Sodium _____

Total Daily Caloric Intake:

Calories _____

Water _____

_____ gms Carb

_____ gms Protein

_____ gms Fat

creating balance

Exercise Journal

Cardio

Type of Cardio: _____

Duration: _____

Intensity: _____

Calories Burned: _____

Type of Cardio: _____

Duration: _____

Intensity: _____

Calories Burned: _____

Weight Training

Type of Exercise: _____
Reps: _____
Sets: _____
Amount of Weight: _____

Type of Exercise: _____
Reps: _____
Sets: _____
Amount of Weight: _____

Type of Exercise: _____
Reps: _____
Sets: _____
Amount of Weight: _____

Type of Exercise: _____
Reps: _____
Sets: _____
Amount of Weight: _____

Type of Exercise: _____
Reps: _____
Sets: _____
Amount of Weight: _____

Self-Assessment Journal

Reflect on the 5 elements of your life. Jot down positive and negative influences and/or experiences of the day. Think about what YOU can do differently to reduce or change the negative and promote more positive. Then put your plan into ACTION!

Spiritual: Did you pray/meditate today? Have you asked for forgiveness for yourself and forgiven others? Have you been grateful and thankful for your blessings? Have you been grateful for the life that has been given to you and do you understand that everything happens for a reason?

Positive

_____

_____

_____

Negative

_____

_____

_____

Plan of Action

_____

_____

_____

Emotional: Did you take a moment to yourself in the morning to pay attention to how you felt, before you started your day? Did you express your emotions instead of suppressing them? Did you acknowledge and allow yourself to feel and experience a range of emotions appropriately, without overreacting? Did you understand the emotions that you felt and not allow them to take you to your past?

Positive

Negative

Plan of Action

Physical: Did you take care of yourself today? Did you eat six small meals? Did you exercise? Did you smoke? Did you drink alcohol? Did you eat fast food?

Positive

_____
_____
_____

Negative

_____
_____
_____

Plan of Action

_____
_____
_____

Social: Who were you around socially? How did it make you feel? Did you limit your exposure to negative surroundings and understand what you felt? Did you give in to negative influences?

Positive

Negative

Plan of Action

Intellectual: Did you plan your day out by writing it down? Did you plan ahead to exercise? Did you prepare your meals and healthy snacks? Did you skip breakfast because you were rushing to work? Did you choose an unhealthy snack because you didn't prepare? Don't forget

Positive

_____
_____
_____

Negative

_____
_____
_____

Plan of Action

_____
_____
_____

creating balance

Meal Journal

Day 3   Date: _____

Quote of the Day: The only way this word can survive is to heal the people. Then people can heal the world because they are the ones who inflicted the problems and pain. The more we destroy nature, the more we destroy a part of ourselves because God made all. The one way to true happiness is to reclaim our childhood by eliminating all things that were introduced to us in our adulthood, for example: worry, greed, doubt, junk, TV, alcohol, drugs, and material things.

Meal 1   Time _____

_____

_____

_____

Water _____

Protein _____

Complex CHO _____

Simple CHO _____

Fat _____

Sodium _____

Meal 2   Time _____

_____

_____

_____

Water _____

Protein _____

Complex CHO _____

Simple CHO _____

Fat _____

Sodium _____

Meal 3   Time _____

_____

_____

_____

Water _____

Protein _____

Complex CHO _____

Simple CHO _____

Fat _____

Sodium _____

Meal 4   Time _____

_____

_____

_____

Water _____

Protein _____

Complex CHO _____

Simple CHO _____

Fat _____

Sodium _____

Meal 5   Time _____

_____

_____

_____

Water _____

Protein _____

Complex CHO _____

Simple CHO _____

Fat _____

Sodium _____

Meal 6   Time _____

_____

_____

_____

Water _____

Protein _____

Complex CHO _____

Simple CHO _____

Fat _____

Sodium _____

Total Daily Caloric Intake:

Calories _____

Water _____

_____ gms Carb

_____ gms Protein

_____ gms Fat

creating balance

Exercise Journal

Cardio

Type of Cardio: _____

Duration: _____

Intensity: _____

Calories Burned: _____

Type of Cardio: _____

Duration: _____

Intensity: _____

Calories Burned: _____

Weight Training

Type of Exercise: _____

Reps: _____

Sets: _____

Amount of Weight: _____

Type of Exercise: _____

Reps: _____

Sets: _____

Amount of Weight: _____

Type of Exercise: _____

Reps: _____

Sets: _____

Amount of Weight: _____

Type of Exercise: _____

Reps: _____

Sets: _____

Amount of Weight: _____

Type of Exercise: _____

Reps: _____

Sets: _____

Amount of Weight: _____

Self-Assessment Journal

Reflect on the 5 elements of your life. Jot down positive and negative influences and/or experiences of the day. Think about what YOU can do differently to reduce or change the negative and promote more positive. Then put your plan into ACTION!

Spiritual: Did you pray/meditate today? Have you asked for forgiveness for yourself and forgiven others? Have you been grateful and thankful for your blessings? Have you been grateful for the life that has been given to you and do you understand that everything happens for a reason?

Positive

_____

_____

_____

Negative

_____

_____

_____

Plan of Action

_____

_____

_____

Emotional: Did you take a moment to yourself in the morning to pay attention to how you felt, before you started your day? Did you express your emotions instead of suppressing them? Did you acknowledge and allow yourself to feel and experience a range of emotions appropriately, without overreacting? Did you understand the emotions that you felt and not allow them to take you to your past?

Positive

Negative

Plan of Action

Physical: Did you take care of yourself today? Did you eat six small meals? Did you exercise? Did you smoke? Did you drink alcohol? Did you eat fast food?

Positive

_____
_____
_____

Negative

_____
_____
_____

Plan of Action

_____
_____
_____

Social: Who were you around socially? How did it make you feel? Did you limit your exposure to negative surroundings and understand what you felt? Did you give in to negative influences?

Positive

___
___
___

Negative

___
___
___

Plan of Action

___
___
___

Intellectual: Did you plan your day out by writing it down? Did you plan ahead to exercise? Did you prepare your meals and healthy snacks? Did you skip breakfast because you were rushing to work? Did you choose an unhealthy snack because you didn't prepare? Don't forget

Positive

_____
_____
_____

Negative

_____
_____
_____

Plan of Action

_____
_____
_____

creating balance

Three Things to Remember

It takes three days for the body to recognize change.

In three weeks, we create habits, remember, first three days are important.

It takes three months for gains in your fitness and life goals, whatever it may be.

Life is a Journey

When you journey the wrong way and it seems hard, you end up lost. But once you find the right way, you can see your goal clearly and it is a much easier way.

Weight Train: two to three days per week; strong, feel

Cardio: three to five days per week for fat loss

Eat: four to six small meals per day, i.e., fat: 3-8 grams, protein: 15-30 grams, carbs: 20-50 grams, per meal.

Flexibility: Stretch three to five times per week for 15-20 minutes per day, hold for about 15-30 seconds each; sense of well-being and injury prevention.

These are the tools! Go For it!!!

A.M. Total Being Fitness

Meal Journal

Day 4   Date: _____

Quote of the Day: *Your body has to have the right kind of fuel and most move 80 percent of the time and be challenged. Emotions must be acted out or talked about, not held in. If you have anger, fear, sadness, happiness, etc., it must be animated and acted out (within reason) in order to have a clear mind. Things that have to be done, such as cleaning your house, going to the bank, etc., must be acted out to clear your mind!*

Meal 1   Time _____   Protein _____

_____   Complex CHO _____

_____   Simple CHO _____

_____   Fat _____

Water _____   Sodium _____

Meal 2   Time _____   Protein _____

_____   Complex CHO _____

_____   Simple CHO _____

_____   Fat _____

Water _____   Sodium _____

Meal 3   Time _____   Protein _____

_____   Complex CHO _____

_____   Simple CHO _____

_____   Fat _____

Water _____   Sodium _____

Meal 4   Time _____

_____

_____

_____

Water _____

Protein _____

Complex CHO _____

Simple CHO _____

Fat _____

Sodium _____

Meal 5   Time _____

_____

_____

_____

Water _____

Protein _____

Complex CHO _____

Simple CHO _____

Fat _____

Sodium _____

Meal 6   Time _____

_____

_____

_____

Water _____

Protein _____

Complex CHO _____

Simple CHO _____

Fat _____

Sodium _____

Total Daily Caloric Intake:

Calories _____

Water _____

_____ gms Carb

_____ gms Protein

_____ gms Fat

Exercise Journal

Cardio

Type of Cardio: _____

Duration: _____

Intensity: _____

Calories Burned: _____

Type of Cardio: _____

Duration: _____

Intensity: _____

Calories Burned: _____

Weight Training

Type of Exercise: _____

Reps: _____

Sets: _____

Amount of Weight: _____

Type of Exercise: _____

Reps: _____

Sets: _____

Amount of Weight: _____

Type of Exercise: _____

Reps: _____

Sets: _____

Amount of Weight: _____

Type of Exercise: _____

Reps: _____

Sets: _____

Amount of Weight: _____

Type of Exercise: _____

Reps: _____

Sets: _____

Amount of Weight: _____

creating balance

Self-Assessment Journal

Reflect on the 5 elements of your life. Jot down positive and negative influences and/or experiences of the day. Think about what YOU can do differently to reduce or change the negative and promote more positive. Then put your plan into ACTION!

Spiritual: Did you pray/meditate today? Have you asked for forgiveness for yourself and forgiven others? Have you been grateful and thankful for your blessings? Have you been grateful for the life that has been given to you and do you understand that everything happens for a reason?

Positive

_____

_____

_____

Negative

_____

_____

_____

Plan of Action

_____

_____

_____

Emotional: Did you take a moment to yourself in the morning to pay attention to how you felt, before you started your day? Did you express your emotions instead of suppressing them? Did you acknowledge and allow yourself to feel and experience a range of emotions appropriately, without overreacting? Did you understand the emotions that you felt and not allow them to take you to your past?

Positive

_____
_____
_____

Negative

_____
_____
_____

Plan of Action

_____
_____
_____

Physical: Did you take care of yourself today? Did you eat six small meals? Did you exercise? Did you smoke? Did you drink alcohol? Did you eat fast food?

Positive

___

___

___

Negative

___

___

___

Plan of Action

___

___

___

Social: Who were you around socially? How did it make you feel? Did you limit your exposure to negative surroundings and understand what you felt? Did you give in to negative influences?

Positive

_____
_____
_____

Negative

_____
_____
_____

Plan of Action

_____
_____
_____

Intellectual: Did you plan your day out by writing it down? Did you plan ahead to exercise? Did you prepare your meals and healthy snacks? Did you skip breakfast because you were rushing to work? Did you choose an unhealthy snack because you didn't prepare? Don't forget

Positive

Negative

Plan of Action

A.M. Total Being Fitness

Meal Journal

Day 5   Date: _____

Quote of the Day: *Life is a Journey. When you travel the wrong way, you end up lost and life seems hard. But once you find the right way, you can see your path clearly and your life becomes much easier and your goals are reached.*

Meal 1   Time _____

_____

_____

_____

Water _____

Protein _____

Complex CHO _____

Simple CHO _____

Fat _____

Sodium _____

Meal 2   Time _____

_____

_____

_____

Water _____

Protein _____

Complex CHO _____

Simple CHO _____

Fat _____

Sodium _____

Meal 3   Time _____

_____

_____

_____

Water _____

Protein _____

Complex CHO _____

Simple CHO _____

Fat _____

Sodium _____

Meal 4   Time _____

_____

_____

_____

Water _____

Protein _____

Complex CHO _____

Simple CHO _____

Fat _____

Sodium _____

Meal 5   Time _____

_____

_____

_____

Water _____

Protein _____

Complex CHO _____

Simple CHO _____

Fat _____

Sodium _____

Meal 6   Time _____

_____

_____

_____

Water _____

Protein _____

Complex CHO _____

Simple CHO _____

Fat _____

Sodium _____

Total Daily Caloric Intake:

Calories _____

Water _____

_____ gms Carb

_____ gms Protein

_____ gms Fat

A.M. Total Being Fitness

Exercise Journal

Cardio

Type of Cardio: _____

Duration: _____

Intensity: _____

Calories Burned: _____

Type of Cardio: _____

Duration: _____

Intensity: _____

Calories Burned: _____

Weight Training

Type of Exercise: _____

Reps: _____

Sets: _____

Amount of Weight: _____

Type of Exercise: _____

Reps: _____

Sets: _____

Amount of Weight: _____

Type of Exercise: _____

Reps: _____

Sets: _____

Amount of Weight: _____

Type of Exercise: _____

Reps: _____

Sets: _____

Amount of Weight: _____

Type of Exercise: _____

Reps: _____

Sets: _____

Amount of Weight: _____

creating balance

Self-Assessment Journal

Reflect on the 5 elements of your life. Jot down positive and negative influences and/or experiences of the day. Think about what YOU can do differently to reduce or change the negative and promote more positive. Then put your plan into ACTION!

Spiritual: Did you pray/meditate today? Have you asked for forgiveness for yourself and forgiven others? Have you been grateful and thankful for your blessings? Have you been grateful for the life that has been given to you and do you understand that everything happens for a reason?

Positive

_____

_____

_____

Negative

_____

_____

_____

Plan of Action

_____

_____

_____

Emotional: Did you take a moment to yourself in the morning to pay attention to how you felt, before you started your day? Did you express your emotions instead of suppressing them? Did you acknowledge and allow yourself to feel and experience a range of emotions appropriately, without overreacting? Did you understand the emotions that you felt and not allow them to take you to your past?

Positive

_____
_____
_____

Negative

_____
_____
_____

Plan of Action

_____
_____
_____

Physical: Did you take care of yourself today? Did you eat six small meals? Did you exercise? Did you smoke? Did you drink alcohol? Did you eat fast food?

Positive

___

___

___

Negative

___

___

___

Plan of Action

___

___

___

Social: Who were you around socially? How did it make you feel? Did you limit your exposure to negative surroundings and understand what you felt? Did you give in to negative influences?

Positive

_____
_____
_____

Negative

_____
_____
_____

Plan of Action

_____
_____
_____

Intellectual: Did you plan your day out by writing it down? Did you plan ahead to exercise? Did you prepare your meals and healthy snacks? Did you skip breakfast because you were rushing to work? Did you choose an unhealthy snack because you didn't prepare? Don't forget

Positive

Negative

Plan of Action

A.M. Total Being Fitness

Meal Journal

Day 6   Date: _____

Quote of the Day: **RELATIONSHIPS.** *When we first meet someone, we try to understand them. But what we don't understand is that when we meet someone, we are not adapting to just that person. We are adapting to their parents, siblings, social habits, and spiritual beliefs. Once we emotionally understand these things and see with our hearts, not with our eyes, we can then grow with this person.*

Meal 1   Time _____

_____

_____

_____

Water _____

Protein _____

Complex CHO _____

Simple CHO _____

Fat _____

Sodium _____

Meal 2   Time _____

_____

_____

_____

Water _____

Protein _____

Complex CHO _____

Simple CHO _____

Fat _____

Sodium _____

Meal 3   Time _____

_____

_____

_____

Water _____

Protein _____

Complex CHO _____

Simple CHO _____

Fat _____

Sodium _____

Meal 4   Time _____

_____

_____

_____

Water _____

Protein _____

Complex CHO _____

Simple CHO _____

Fat _____

Sodium _____

Meal 5   Time _____

_____

_____

_____

Water _____

Protein _____

Complex CHO _____

Simple CHO _____

Fat _____

Sodium _____

Meal 6   Time _____

_____

_____

_____

Water _____

Protein _____

Complex CHO _____

Simple CHO _____

Fat _____

Sodium _____

Total Daily Caloric Intake:

Calories _____

Water _____

_____ gms Carb

_____ gms Protein

_____ gms Fat

Exercise Journal

Cardio

Type of Cardio: _____

Duration: _____

Intensity: _____

Calories Burned: _____

Type of Cardio: _____

Duration: _____

Intensity: _____

Calories Burned: _____

Weight Training

Type of Exercise: _____

Reps: _____

Sets: _____

Amount of Weight: _____

Type of Exercise: _____

Reps: _____

Sets: _____

Amount of Weight: _____

Type of Exercise: _____

Reps: _____

Sets: _____

Amount of Weight: _____

Type of Exercise: _____

Reps: _____

Sets: _____

Amount of Weight: _____

Type of Exercise: _____

Reps: _____

Sets: _____

Amount of Weight: _____

Self-Assessment Journal

Reflect on the 5 elements of your life. Jot down positive and negative influences and/or experiences of the day. Think about what YOU can do differently to reduce or change the negative and promote more positive. Then put your plan into ACTION!

Spiritual: Did you pray/meditate today? Have you asked for forgiveness for yourself and forgiven others? Have you been grateful and thankful for your blessings? Have you been grateful for the life that has been given to you and do you understand that everything happens for a reason?

Positive

_____

_____

_____

Negative

_____

_____

_____

Plan of Action

_____

_____

_____

Emotional: Did you take a moment to yourself in the morning to pay attention to how you felt, before you started your day? Did you express your emotions instead of suppressing them? Did you acknowledge and allow yourself to feel and experience a range of emotions appropriately, without overreacting? Did you understand the emotions that you felt and not allow them to take you to your past?

Positive

_____

_____

_____

Negative

_____

_____

_____

Plan of Action

_____

_____

_____

Physical: Did you take care of yourself today? Did you eat six small meals? Did you exercise? Did you smoke? Did you drink alcohol? Did you eat fast food?

Positive

___

___

___

Negative

___

___

___

Plan of Action

___

___

___

Social: Who were you around socially? How did it make you feel? Did you limit your exposure to negative surroundings and understand what you felt? Did you give in to negative influences?

Positive

_____
_____
_____

Negative

_____
_____
_____

Plan of Action

_____
_____
_____

Intellectual: Did you plan your day out by writing it down? Did you plan ahead to exercise? Did you prepare your meals and healthy snacks? Did you skip breakfast because you were rushing to work? Did you choose an unhealthy snack because you didn't prepare? Don't forget

Positive

_____
_____
_____

Negative

_____
_____
_____

Plan of Action

_____
_____
_____

A.M. Total Being Fitness

Meal Journal

Day 7   Date: _____

Quote of the Day: *People are put in our lives for a reason. Just like the sun, the birds, and the plants. Everything on this Earth needs something in order to survive, especially people. People need to give one another therapy with Love and Understanding.*

Meal 1   Time _____

_____

_____

_____

Water _____

Protein _____

Complex CHO _____

Simple CHO _____

Fat _____

Sodium _____

Meal 2   Time _____

_____

_____

_____

Water _____

Protein _____

Complex CHO _____

Simple CHO _____

Fat _____

Sodium _____

Meal 3   Time _____

_____

_____

_____

Water _____

Protein _____

Complex CHO _____

Simple CHO _____

Fat _____

Sodium _____

Meal 4   Time _____

_____

_____

_____

Water _____

Protein _____

Complex CHO _____

Simple CHO _____

Fat _____

Sodium _____

Meal 5   Time _____

_____

_____

_____

Water _____

Protein _____

Complex CHO _____

Simple CHO _____

Fat _____

Sodium _____

Meal 6   Time _____

_____

_____

_____

Water _____

Protein _____

Complex CHO _____

Simple CHO _____

Fat _____

Sodium _____

Total Daily Caloric Intake:

Calories _____

Water _____

_____gms Carb

_____ gms Protein

_____gms Fat

Exercise Journal

Cardio

Type of Cardio: _____

Duration: _____

Intensity: _____

Calories Burned: _____

Type of Cardio: _____

Duration: _____

Intensity: _____

Calories Burned: _____

Weight Training

Type of Exercise: _____

Reps: _____

Sets: _____

Amount of Weight: _____

Type of Exercise: _____

Reps: _____

Sets: _____

Amount of Weight: _____

Type of Exercise: _____

Reps: _____

Sets: _____

Amount of Weight: _____

Type of Exercise: _____

Reps: _____

Sets: _____

Amount of Weight: _____

Type of Exercise: _____

Reps: _____

Sets: _____

Amount of Weight: _____

creating balance

Self-Assessment Journal

Reflect on the 5 elements of your life. Jot down positive and negative influences and/or experiences of the day. Think about what YOU can do differently to reduce or change the negative and promote more positive. Then put your plan into ACTION!

Spiritual: Did you pray/meditate today? Have you asked for forgiveness for yourself and forgiven others? Have you been grateful and thankful for your blessings? Have you been grateful for the life that has been given to you and do you understand that everything happens for a reason?

Positive

Negative

Plan of Action

Emotional: Did you take a moment to yourself in the morning to pay attention to how you felt, before you started your day? Did you express your emotions instead of suppressing them? Did you acknowledge and allow yourself to feel and experience a range of emotions appropriately, without overreacting? Did you understand the emotions that you felt and not allow them to take you to your past?

Positive

_____

_____

_____

Negative

_____

_____

_____

Plan of Action

_____

_____

_____

Physical: Did you take care of yourself today? Did you eat six small meals? Did you exercise? Did you smoke? Did you drink alcohol? Did you eat fast food?

Positive

Negative

Plan of Action

Social: Who were you around socially? How did it make you feel? Did you limit your exposure to negative surroundings and understand what you felt? Did you give in to negative influences?

Positive

___

___

___

Negative

___

___

___

Plan of Action

___

___

___

Intellectual: Did you plan your day out by writing it down? Did you plan ahead to exercise? Did you prepare your meals and healthy snacks? Did you skip breakfast because you were rushing to work? Did you choose an unhealthy snack because you didn't prepare? Don't forget

Positive

Negative

Plan of Action

Picture this...

You are a producer and the main character in a movie called "Life."

You aren't happy with your role.

You desire to change your image.

Lights! Just as lighting on a set can change how things look, so can we change our "image." Through weight training, we firm up and sculpt muscles, which improve our appearance and how we feel.

Camera! When we eat healthier, we feel better. When we feel better, out outlook or "angle" on life also changes for the best.

Action! When we exercise, our "action" creates a reaction – no only a stronger, healthier body, but also an overall positive lifestyle. Reaching our goals and true destination is the "climax" of your movie.

Put them all together and you have a great "production," called A Balanced Life!

creating balance

Meal Journal

Day 8   Date: _____

Quote of the Day: *What is failure? Why is it important?*
Without failure we cannot appreciate our accomplishments!

Meal 1   Time _____

_____

_____

_____

Water _____

Protein _____

Complex CHO _____

Simple CHO _____

Fat _____

Sodium _____

Meal 2   Time _____

_____

_____

_____

Water _____

Protein _____

Complex CHO _____

Simple CHO _____

Fat _____

Sodium _____

Meal 3   Time _____

_____

_____

_____

Water _____

Protein _____

Complex CHO _____

Simple CHO _____

Fat _____

Sodium _____

Meal 4   Time _____

_____

_____

_____

Water _____

Protein _____

Complex CHO _____

Simple CHO _____

Fat _____

Sodium _____

Meal 5   Time _____

_____

_____

_____

Water _____

Protein _____

Complex CHO _____

Simple CHO _____

Fat _____

Sodium _____

Meal 6   Time _____

_____

_____

_____

Water _____

Protein _____

Complex CHO _____

Simple CHO _____

Fat _____

Sodium _____

Total Daily Caloric Intake:

Calories _____

Water _____

_____ gms Carb

_____ gms Protein

_____ gms Fat

creating balance

Exercise Journal

Cardio

Type of Cardio: _____

Duration: _____

Intensity: _____

Calories Burned: _____

Type of Cardio: _____

Duration: _____

Intensity: _____

Calories Burned: _____

Weight Training

Type of Exercise: _____

Reps: _____

Sets: _____

Amount of Weight: _____

Type of Exercise: _____

Reps: _____

Sets: _____

Amount of Weight: _____

Type of Exercise: _____

Reps: _____

Sets: _____

Amount of Weight: _____

Type of Exercise: _____

Reps: _____

Sets: _____

Amount of Weight: _____

Type of Exercise: _____

Reps: _____

Sets: _____

Amount of Weight: _____

Self-Assessment Journal

Reflect on the 5 elements of your life. Jot down positive and negative influences and/or experiences of the day. Think about what YOU can do differently to reduce or change the negative and promote more positive. Then put your plan into ACTION!

Spiritual: Did you pray/meditate today? Have you asked for forgiveness for yourself and forgiven others? Have you been grateful and thankful for your blessings? Have you been grateful for the life that has been given to you and do you understand that everything happens for a reason?

Positive

_____

_____

_____

Negative

_____

_____

_____

Plan of Action

_____

_____

_____

Emotional: Did you take a moment to yourself in the morning to pay attention to how you felt, before you started your day? Did you express your emotions instead of suppressing them? Did you acknowledge and allow yourself to feel and experience a range of emotions appropriately, without overreacting? Did you understand the emotions that you felt and not allow them to take you to your past?

Positive

___

___

___

Negative

___

___

___

Plan of Action

___

___

___

Physical: Did you take care of yourself today? Did you eat six small meals? Did you exercise? Did you smoke? Did you drink alcohol? Did you eat fast food?

Positive

_____
_____
_____

Negative

_____
_____
_____

Plan of Action

_____
_____
_____

Social: Who were you around socially? How did it make you feel? Did you limit your exposure to negative surroundings and understand what you felt? Did you give in to negative influences?

Positive

___

___

___

Negative

___

___

___

Plan of Action

___

___

___

Intellectual: Did you plan your day out by writing it down? Did you plan ahead to exercise? Did you prepare your meals and healthy snacks? Did you skip breakfast because you were rushing to work? Did you choose an unhealthy snack because you didn't prepare? Don't forget

Positive

_____
_____
_____

Negative

_____
_____
_____

Plan of Action

_____
_____
_____

creating balance

Meal Journal

Day 9   Date: _____

Quote of the Day: *The door to our mind is our ears.*
The door to our eyes is our body. The door to our soul is our heart!

Meal 1   Time _____

_____

_____

_____

Water _____

Protein _____

Complex CHO _____

Simple CHO _____

Fat _____

Sodium _____

Meal 2   Time _____

_____

_____

_____

Water _____

Protein _____

Complex CHO _____

Simple CHO _____

Fat _____

Sodium _____

Meal 3   Time _____

_____

_____

_____

Water _____

Protein _____

Complex CHO _____

Simple CHO _____

Fat _____

Sodium _____

Meal 4 Time _____

_____

_____

_____

Water _____

Protein _____

Complex CHO _____

Simple CHO _____

Fat _____

Sodium _____

Meal 5 Time _____

_____

_____

_____

Water _____

Protein _____

Complex CHO _____

Simple CHO _____

Fat _____

Sodium _____

Meal 6 Time _____

_____

_____

_____

Water _____

Protein _____

Complex CHO _____

Simple CHO _____

Fat _____

Sodium _____

Total Daily Caloric Intake:

Calories _____

Water _____

_____ gms Carb

_____ gms Protein

_____ gms Fat

creating balance

Exercise Journal

Cardio

Type of Cardio: _____

Duration: _____

Intensity: _____

Calories Burned: _____

Type of Cardio: _____

Duration: _____

Intensity: _____

Calories Burned: _____

Weight Training

Type of Exercise: _____

Reps: _____

Sets: _____

Amount of Weight: _____

Type of Exercise: _____

Reps: _____

Sets: _____

Amount of Weight: _____

Type of Exercise: _____

Reps: _____

Sets: _____

Amount of Weight: _____

Type of Exercise: _____

Reps: _____

Sets: _____

Amount of Weight: _____

Type of Exercise: _____

Reps: _____

Sets: _____

Amount of Weight: _____

Self-Assessment Journal

Reflect on the 5 elements of your life. Jot down positive and negative influences and/or experiences of the day. Think about what YOU can do differently to reduce or change the negative and promote more positive. Then put your plan into ACTION!

Spiritual: Did you pray/meditate today? Have you asked for forgiveness for yourself and forgiven others? Have you been grateful and thankful for your blessings? Have you been grateful for the life that has been given to you and do you understand that everything happens for a reason?

Positive

Negative

Plan of Action

Emotional: Did you take a moment to yourself in the morning to pay attention to how you felt, before you started your day? Did you express your emotions instead of suppressing them? Did you acknowledge and allow yourself to feel and experience a range of emotions appropriately, without overreacting? Did you understand the emotions that you felt and not allow them to take you to your past?

Positive

Negative

Plan of Action

Physical: Did you take care of yourself today? Did you eat six small meals? Did you exercise? Did you smoke? Did you drink alcohol? Did you eat fast food?

Positive

_____
_____
_____

Negative

_____
_____
_____

Plan of Action

_____
_____
_____

Social: Who were you around socially? How did it make you feel? Did you limit your exposure to negative surroundings and understand what you felt? Did you give in to negative influences?

Positive

___

___

___

Negative

___

___

___

Plan of Action

___

___

___

Intellectual: Did you plan your day out by writing it down? Did you plan ahead to exercise? Did you prepare your meals and healthy snacks? Did you skip breakfast because you were rushing to work? Did you choose an unhealthy snack because you didn't prepare? Don't forget

Positive

_____

_____

_____

Negative

_____

_____

_____

Plan of Action

_____

_____

_____

creating balance

Meal Journal

Day 10   Date: _____

Quote of the Day: *Remember, every fault an adult has was learned in childhood. Every fault a child has was learned from an adult. So, take a good look at yourself! Forgive and try to understand others.*

Meal 1   Time _____

_____

_____

_____

Water _____

Protein _____

Complex CHO _____

Simple CHO _____

Fat _____

Sodium _____

Meal 2   Time _____

_____

_____

_____

Water _____

Protein _____

Complex CHO _____

Simple CHO _____

Fat _____

Sodium _____

Meal 3   Time _____

_____

_____

_____

Water _____

Protein _____

Complex CHO _____

Simple CHO _____

Fat _____

Sodium _____

Meal 4   Time _____

_____

_____

_____

Water _____

Protein _____

Complex CHO _____

Simple CHO _____

Fat _____

Sodium _____

Meal 5   Time _____

_____

_____

_____

Water _____

Protein _____

Complex CHO _____

Simple CHO _____

Fat _____

Sodium _____

Meal 6   Time _____

_____

_____

_____

Water _____

Protein _____

Complex CHO _____

Simple CHO _____

Fat _____

Sodium _____

Total Daily Caloric Intake:

Calories _____

Water _____

_____ gms Carb

_____ gms Protein

_____ gms Fat

creating balance

Exercise Journal

Cardio

Type of Cardio: _____

Duration: _____

Intensity: _____

Calories Burned: _____

Type of Cardio: _____

Duration: _____

Intensity: _____

Calories Burned: _____

Weight Training

Type of Exercise: _____

Reps: _____

Sets: _____

Amount of Weight: _____

Type of Exercise: _____

Reps: _____

Sets: _____

Amount of Weight: _____

Type of Exercise: _____

Reps: _____

Sets: _____

Amount of Weight: _____

Type of Exercise: _____

Reps: _____

Sets: _____

Amount of Weight: _____

Type of Exercise: _____

Reps: _____

Sets: _____

Amount of Weight: _____

A.M. Total Being Fitness

Self-Assessment Journal

Reflect on the 5 elements of your life. Jot down positive and negative influences and/or experiences of the day. Think about what YOU can do differently to reduce or change the negative and promote more positive. Then put your plan into ACTION!

Spiritual: Did you pray/meditate today? Have you asked for forgiveness for yourself and forgiven others? Have you been grateful and thankful for your blessings? Have you been grateful for the life that has been given to you and do you understand that everything happens for a reason?

Positive

_____

_____

_____

Negative

_____

_____

_____

Plan of Action

_____

_____

_____

Emotional: Did you take a moment to yourself in the morning to pay attention to how you felt, before you started your day? Did you express your emotions instead of suppressing them? Did you acknowledge and allow yourself to feel and experience a range of emotions appropriately, without overreacting? Did you understand the emotions that you felt and not allow them to take you to your past?

Positive

Negative

Plan of Action

Physical: Did you take care of yourself today? Did you eat six small meals? Did you exercise? Did you smoke? Did you drink alcohol? Did you eat fast food?

Positive

_____
_____
_____

Negative

_____
_____
_____

Plan of Action

_____
_____
_____

Social: Who were you around socially? How did it make you feel? Did you limit your exposure to negative surroundings and understand what you felt? Did you give in to negative influences?

Positive

Negative

Plan of Action

Intellectual: Did you plan your day out by writing it down? Did you plan ahead to exercise? Did you prepare your meals and healthy snacks? Did you skip breakfast because you were rushing to work? Did you choose an unhealthy snack because you didn't prepare? Don't forget

Positive

_____

_____

_____

Negative

_____

_____

_____

Plan of Action

_____

_____

_____

Just go with the flow

Spring time, it is our time for
birth and planning, this
would be.
The dawn.

Summer time. Is our time
growth and expanding
intense focus, this
is the mid-morning.

Autumn time. Is our time to
harvest what we have
accumulated,
this is mid-pm.

Winter time. Is time for
storage and rest,
this is the dark-hour.

A.M. Total Being Fitness

Meal Journal

Day 11   Date: _____

Quote of the Day: *Only when we face our problems can we begin to solve them. When we avoid our problems, we feel stress from them.*

Meal 1   Time _____
_____
_____
_____
Water _____

Protein _____
Complex CHO _____
Simple CHO _____
Fat _____
Sodium _____

Meal 2   Time _____
_____
_____
_____
Water _____

Protein _____
Complex CHO _____
Simple CHO _____
Fat _____
Sodium _____

Meal 3   Time _____
_____
_____
_____
Water _____

Protein _____
Complex CHO _____
Simple CHO _____
Fat _____
Sodium _____

Meal 4   Time _____   Protein _____

_____   Complex CHO _____

_____   Simple CHO _____

_____   Fat _____

Water _____   Sodium _____

Meal 5   Time _____   Protein _____

_____   Complex CHO _____

_____   Simple CHO _____

_____   Fat _____

Water _____   Sodium _____

Meal 6   Time _____   Protein _____

_____   Complex CHO _____

_____   Simple CHO _____

_____   Fat _____

Water _____   Sodium _____

Total Daily Caloric Intake:

Calories _____

Water _____

_____ gms Carb

_____ gms Protein

_____ gms Fat

A.M. Total Being Fitness

Exercise Journal

Cardio

Type of Cardio: _____

Duration: _____

Intensity: _____

Calories Burned: _____

Type of Cardio: _____

Duration: _____

Intensity: _____

Calories Burned: _____

Weight Training

Type of Exercise: _____

Reps: _____

Sets: _____

Amount of Weight: _____

Type of Exercise: _____

Reps: _____

Sets: _____

Amount of Weight: _____

Type of Exercise: _____

Reps: _____

Sets: _____

Amount of Weight: _____

Type of Exercise: _____

Reps: _____

Sets: _____

Amount of Weight: _____

Type of Exercise: _____

Reps: _____

Sets: _____

Amount of Weight: _____

creating balance

Self-Assessment Journal

Reflect on the 5 elements of your life. Jot down positive and negative influences and/or experiences of the day. Think about what YOU can do differently to reduce or change the negative and promote more positive. Then put your plan into ACTION!

Spiritual: Did you pray/meditate today? Have you asked for forgiveness for yourself and forgiven others? Have you been grateful and thankful for your blessings? Have you been grateful for the life that has been given to you and do you understand that everything happens for a reason?

Positive

_____

_____

_____

Negative

_____

_____

_____

Plan of Action

_____

_____

_____

Emotional: Did you take a moment to yourself in the morning to pay attention to how you felt, before you started your day? Did you express your emotions instead of suppressing them? Did you acknowledge and allow yourself to feel and experience a range of emotions appropriately, without overreacting? Did you understand the emotions that you felt and not allow them to take you to your past?

Positive

_____
_____
_____

Negative

_____
_____
_____

Plan of Action

_____
_____
_____

Physical: Did you take care of yourself today? Did you eat six small meals? Did you exercise? Did you smoke? Did you drink alcohol? Did you eat fast food?

Positive

_____
_____
_____

Negative

_____
_____
_____

Plan of Action

_____
_____
_____

Social: Who were you around socially? How did it make you feel? Did you limit your exposure to negative surroundings and understand what you felt? Did you give in to negative influences?

Positive

___
___
___

Negative

___
___
___

Plan of Action

___
___
___

Intellectual: Did you plan your day out by writing it down? Did you plan ahead to exercise? Did you prepare your meals and healthy snacks? Did you skip breakfast because you were rushing to work? Did you choose an unhealthy snack because you didn't prepare? Don't forget

Positive

Negative

Plan of Action

A.M. Total Being Fitness

Meal Journal

Day 12   Date: _____

Quote of the Day: Stop! *Look in the mirror! No, look a little deeper! What we see when we focus on the outside is what we bring inside of us, and that is what we become. But when we focus from the inside, we can then change our outside appearance.*

Meal 1   Time _____

_____

_____

_____

Water _____

Protein _____

Complex CHO _____

Simple CHO _____

Fat _____

Sodium _____

Meal 2   Time _____

_____

_____

_____

Water _____

Protein _____

Complex CHO _____

Simple CHO _____

Fat _____

Sodium _____

Meal 3   Time _____

_____

_____

_____

Water _____

Protein _____

Complex CHO _____

Simple CHO _____

Fat _____

Sodium _____

creating balance

Meal 4 Time _____

_____

_____

_____

Water _____

Protein _____

Complex CHO _____

Simple CHO _____

Fat _____

Sodium _____

Meal 5 Time _____

_____

_____

_____

Water _____

Protein _____

Complex CHO _____

Simple CHO _____

Fat _____

Sodium _____

Meal 6 Time _____

_____

_____

_____

Water _____

Protein _____

Complex CHO _____

Simple CHO _____

Fat _____

Sodium _____

Total Daily Caloric Intake:

Calories _____

Water _____

_____ gms Carb

_____ gms Protein

_____ gms Fat

Exercise Journal

Cardio

Type of Cardio: _____

Duration: _____

Intensity: _____

Calories Burned: _____

Type of Cardio: _____

Duration: _____

Intensity: _____

Calories Burned: _____

Weight Training

Type of Exercise: _____

Reps: _____

Sets: _____

Amount of Weight: _____

Type of Exercise: _____

Reps: _____

Sets: _____

Amount of Weight: _____

Type of Exercise: _____

Reps: _____

Sets: _____

Amount of Weight: _____

Type of Exercise: _____

Reps: _____

Sets: _____

Amount of Weight: _____

Type of Exercise: _____

Reps: _____

Sets: _____

Amount of Weight: _____

Self-Assessment Journal

Reflect on the 5 elements of your life. Jot down positive and negative influences and/or experiences of the day. Think about what YOU can do differently to reduce or change the negative and promote more positive. Then put your plan into ACTION!

Spiritual: Did you pray/meditate today? Have you asked for forgiveness for yourself and forgiven others? Have you been grateful and thankful for your blessings? Have you been grateful for the life that has been given to you and do you understand that everything happens for a reason?

Positive

_____

_____

_____

Negative

_____

_____

_____

Plan of Action

_____

_____

_____

Emotional: Did you take a moment to yourself in the morning to pay attention to how you felt, before you started your day? Did you express your emotions instead of suppressing them? Did you acknowledge and allow yourself to feel and experience a range of emotions appropriately, without overreacting? Did you understand the emotions that you felt and not allow them to take you to your past?

Positive

___

___

___

Negative

___

___

___

Plan of Action

___

___

___

Physical: Did you take care of yourself today? Did you eat six small meals? Did you exercise? Did you smoke? Did you drink alcohol? Did you eat fast food?

Positive

Negative

Plan of Action

Social: Who were you around socially? How did it make you feel? Did you limit your exposure to negative surroundings and understand what you felt? Did you give in to negative influences?

Positive

_____

_____

_____

Negative

_____

_____

_____

Plan of Action

_____

_____

_____

Intellectual: Did you plan your day out by writing it down? Did you plan ahead to exercise? Did you prepare your meals and healthy snacks? Did you skip breakfast because you were rushing to work? Did you choose an unhealthy snack because you didn't prepare? Don't forget

Positive

___

___

___

Negative

___

___

___

Plan of Action

___

___

___

A.M. Total Being Fitness

Meal Journal

Day 13   Date: _____

Quote of the Day: *When we look forward to something that makes us happy, we feel happy. When we look back to something that makes us feel sad, we feel sad. If we do not resolve the thing in our past and we look back, we feel that emotion of what we did. Bottom line: to understand your past, be aware of your present and look forward to a positive and optimistic future!*

Meal 1   Time _____   Protein _____

_____   Complex CHO _____

_____   Simple CHO _____

_____   Fat _____

Water _____   Sodium _____

Meal 2   Time _____   Protein _____

_____   Complex CHO _____

_____   Simple CHO _____

_____   Fat _____

Water _____   Sodium _____

Meal 3   Time _____   Protein _____

_____   Complex CHO _____

_____   Simple CHO _____

_____   Fat _____

Water _____   Sodium _____

Meal 4   Time _____

_____

_____

_____

Water _____

Protein _____

Complex CHO _____

Simple CHO _____

Fat _____

Sodium _____

Meal 5   Time _____

_____

_____

_____

Water _____

Protein _____

Complex CHO _____

Simple CHO _____

Fat _____

Sodium _____

Meal 6   Time _____

_____

_____

_____

Water _____

Protein _____

Complex CHO _____

Simple CHO _____

Fat _____

Sodium _____

Total Daily Caloric Intake:

Calories _____

Water _____

_____gms Carb

_____ gms Protein

_____gms Fat

Exercise Journal

Cardio

Type of Cardio: _____

Duration: _____

Intensity: _____

Calories Burned: _____

Type of Cardio: _____

Duration: _____

Intensity: _____

Calories Burned: _____

Weight Training

Type of Exercise: _____

Reps: _____

Sets: _____

Amount of Weight: _____

Type of Exercise: _____

Reps: _____

Sets: _____

Amount of Weight: _____

Type of Exercise: _____

Reps: _____

Sets: _____

Amount of Weight: _____

Type of Exercise: _____

Reps: _____

Sets: _____

Amount of Weight: _____

Type of Exercise: _____

Reps: _____

Sets: _____

Amount of Weight: _____

Self-Assessment Journal

Reflect on the 5 elements of your life. Jot down positive and negative influences and/or experiences of the day. Think about what YOU can do differently to reduce or change the negative and promote more positive. Then put your plan into ACTION!

Spiritual: Did you pray/meditate today? Have you asked for forgiveness for yourself and forgiven others? Have you been grateful and thankful for your blessings? Have you been grateful for the life that has been given to you and do you understand that everything happens for a reason?

Positive

Negative

Plan of Action

Emotional: Did you take a moment to yourself in the morning to pay attention to how you felt, before you started your day? Did you express your emotions instead of suppressing them? Did you acknowledge and allow yourself to feel and experience a range of emotions appropriately, without overreacting? Did you understand the emotions that you felt and not allow them to take you to your past?

Positive

_____

_____

_____

Negative

_____

_____

_____

Plan of Action

_____

_____

_____

Physical: Did you take care of yourself today? Did you eat six small meals? Did you exercise? Did you smoke? Did you drink alcohol? Did you eat fast food?

Positive

Negative

Plan of Action

Social: Who were you around socially? How did it make you feel? Did you limit your exposure to negative surroundings and understand what you felt? Did you give in to negative influences?

Positive

_____
_____
_____

Negative

_____
_____
_____

Plan of Action

_____
_____
_____

Intellectual: Did you plan your day out by writing it down? Did you plan ahead to exercise? Did you prepare your meals and healthy snacks? Did you skip breakfast because you were rushing to work? Did you choose an unhealthy snack because you didn't prepare? Don't forget

Positive

Negative

Plan of Action

A.M. Total Being Fitness

Meal Journal

Day 14   Date: _____

Quote of the Day: *When you are not in touch with your emotions, you may tend to eat more than your body actually needs, because food equals energy and you will eat to get energy! When you are in touch with your emotions, you will tend to burn more energy than your body has! Because energy equals energy and a good workout creates that energy as opposed to trying to get the energy from food!*

Meal 1   Time _____

_____

_____

_____

Water _____

Protein _____

Complex CHO _____

Simple CHO _____

Fat _____

Sodium _____

Meal 2   Time _____

_____

_____

_____

Water _____

Protein _____

Complex CHO _____

Simple CHO _____

Fat _____

Sodium _____

Meal 3   Time _____

_____

_____

_____

Water _____

Protein _____

Complex CHO _____

Simple CHO _____

Fat _____

Sodium _____

Meal 4   Time _____

_____

_____

_____

Water _____

Protein _____

Complex CHO _____

Simple CHO _____

Fat _____

Sodium _____

Meal 5   Time _____

_____

_____

_____

Water _____

Protein _____

Complex CHO _____

Simple CHO _____

Fat _____

Sodium _____

Meal 6   Time _____

_____

_____

_____

Water _____

Protein _____

Complex CHO _____

Simple CHO _____

Fat _____

Sodium _____

Total Daily Caloric Intake:

Calories _____

Water _____

_____gms Carb

_____ gms Protein

_____gms Fat

Exercise Journal

Cardio

Type of Cardio: _____

Duration: _____

Intensity: _____

Calories Burned: _____

Type of Cardio: _____

Duration: _____

Intensity: _____

Calories Burned: _____

Weight Training

Type of Exercise: _____

Reps: _____

Sets: _____

Amount of Weight: _____

Type of Exercise: _____

Reps: _____

Sets: _____

Amount of Weight: _____

Type of Exercise: _____

Reps: _____

Sets: _____

Amount of Weight: _____

Type of Exercise: _____

Reps: _____

Sets: _____

Amount of Weight: _____

Type of Exercise: _____

Reps: _____

Sets: _____

Amount of Weight: _____

creating balance

Self-Assessment Journal

Reflect on the 5 elements of your life. Jot down positive and negative influences and/or experiences of the day. Think about what YOU can do differently to reduce or change the negative and promote more positive. Then put your plan into ACTION!

Spiritual: Did you pray/meditate today? Have you asked for forgiveness for yourself and forgiven others? Have you been grateful and thankful for your blessings? Have you been grateful for the life that has been given to you and do you understand that everything happens for a reason?

Positive

_____

_____

_____

Negative

_____

_____

_____

Plan of Action

_____

_____

_____

Emotional: Did you take a moment to yourself in the morning to pay attention to how you felt, before you started your day? Did you express your emotions instead of suppressing them? Did you acknowledge and allow yourself to feel and experience a range of emotions appropriately, without overreacting? Did you understand the emotions that you felt and not allow them to take you to your past?

Positive

_____

_____

_____

Negative

_____

_____

_____

Plan of Action

_____

_____

_____

Physical: Did you take care of yourself today? Did you eat six small meals? Did you exercise? Did you smoke? Did you drink alcohol? Did you eat fast food?

Positive

_____
_____
_____

Negative

_____
_____
_____

Plan of Action

_____
_____
_____

Social: Who were you around socially? How did it make you feel? Did you limit your exposure to negative surroundings and understand what you felt? Did you give in to negative influences?

Positive

_____
_____
_____

Negative

_____
_____
_____

Plan of Action

_____
_____
_____

Intellectual: Did you plan your day out by writing it down? Did you plan ahead to exercise? Did you prepare your meals and healthy snacks? Did you skip breakfast because you were rushing to work? Did you choose an unhealthy snack because you didn't prepare? Don't forget

Positive

_____
_____
_____

Negative

_____
_____
_____

Plan of Action

_____
_____
_____

Five Elements Check In

You are unique- made up of many components, both internal and external. Each component is interconnected influencing and impacting the other.

Environment- you are affected by what surrounds you. For example, rain and sunshine enables life on earth to grow. A plant will not grow if it does not get enough water or sunlight. You, too, will not grow if you are surrounded by things that prevent your growth.

Spiritual- Your spiritual self is often described as a *belief in a higher being or one's faith*. You can strengthen your spirituality through practicing your religion, prayer and meditation. If you are open minded, your spirituality can be enhanced through life's experiences. For example, when you share the miracle and joy of the birth of a baby or grieve and reflect on the life of someone who dies, you can experience spiritual.

Emotional- your emotions are *how and what you feel*. Expressing laughter or anger allows us to grow just as when we feel pain and cry. Experiencing all emotions is important to personal growth.

Physical- Your physical capability is *what your body is able to do*. When you train, you overload your cardiovascular and respiratory systems. This increases your ability to take in more oxygen which is necessary for your body to function. When you lift weights, you overload your muscles and increase your

Social- You *interact with people* all of the time. When you surround yourself by negative people, you can start to feel negative. You can turn negative experiences into positive ones. For example, if someone takes advantage of you, you need to learn from the experience and your mistakes. This enables you to grow and become wiser.

Intellectual- Your intellectual side is *what you know*. The more you read, the more knowledge you gain. If you are able to apply what you learn and not just know it, you are even further ahead.

creating balance

Meal Journal

Day 15   Date: _____

Quote of the Day: *You are unique, made up of many components, both internal and external. Each component is interconnected, influencing and impacting the other. Be mindful of the 5 Elements of your Life at all times to keep yourself balanced~*

Meal 1   Time _____

_____

_____

_____

Water _____

Protein _____

Complex CHO _____

Simple CHO _____

Fat _____

Sodium _____

Meal 2   Time _____

_____

_____

_____

Water _____

Protein _____

Complex CHO _____

Simple CHO _____

Fat _____

Sodium _____

Meal 3   Time _____

_____

_____

_____

Water _____

Protein _____

Complex CHO _____

Simple CHO _____

Fat _____

Sodium _____

Meal 4   Time _____

_____

_____

_____

Water _____

Protein _____

Complex CHO _____

Simple CHO _____

Fat _____

Sodium _____

Meal 5   Time _____

_____

_____

_____

Water _____

Protein _____

Complex CHO _____

Simple CHO _____

Fat _____

Sodium _____

Meal 6   Time _____

_____

_____

_____

Water _____

Protein _____

Complex CHO _____

Simple CHO _____

Fat _____

Sodium _____

Total Daily Caloric Intake:

Calories _____

Water _____

_____ gms Carb

_____ gms Protein

_____ gms Fat

creating balance

Exercise Journal

Cardio

Type of Cardio: _____

Duration: _____

Intensity: _____

Calories Burned: _____

Type of Cardio: _____

Duration: _____

Intensity: _____

Calories Burned: _____

Weight Training

Type of Exercise: _____
Reps: _____
Sets: _____
Amount of Weight: _____

Type of Exercise: _____
Reps: _____
Sets: _____
Amount of Weight: _____

Type of Exercise: _____
Reps: _____
Sets: _____
Amount of Weight: _____

Type of Exercise: _____
Reps: _____
Sets: _____
Amount of Weight: _____

Type of Exercise: _____
Reps: _____
Sets: _____
Amount of Weight: _____

Self-Assessment Journal

Reflect on the 5 elements of your life. Jot down positive and negative influences and/or experiences of the day. Think about what YOU can do differently to reduce or change the negative and promote more positive. Then put your plan into ACTION!

Spiritual: Did you pray/meditate today? Have you asked for forgiveness for yourself and forgiven others? Have you been grateful and thankful for your blessings? Have you been grateful for the life that has been given to you and do you understand that everything happens for a reason?

Positive

_____

_____

_____

Negative

_____

_____

_____

Plan of Action

_____

_____

_____

Emotional: Did you take a moment to yourself in the morning to pay attention to how you felt, before you started your day? Did you express your emotions instead of suppressing them? Did you acknowledge and allow yourself to feel and experience a range of emotions appropriately, without overreacting? Did you understand the emotions that you felt and not allow them to take you to your past?

Positive

Negative

Plan of Action

Physical: Did you take care of yourself today? Did you eat six small meals? Did you exercise? Did you smoke? Did you drink alcohol? Did you eat fast food?

Positive

_____
_____
_____

Negative

_____
_____
_____

Plan of Action

_____
_____
_____

Social: Who were you around socially? How did it make you feel? Did you limit your exposure to negative surroundings and understand what you felt? Did you give in to negative influences?

Positive

Negative

Plan of Action

Intellectual: Did you plan your day out by writing it down? Did you plan ahead to exercise? Did you prepare your meals and healthy snacks? Did you skip breakfast because you were rushing to work? Did you choose an unhealthy snack because you didn't prepare? Don't forget

Positive

_____
_____
_____

Negative

_____
_____
_____

Plan of Action

_____
_____
_____

creating balance

Consider This:

10 Easy Steps: Going Back to Our Childhood

Age 0-2

1   We ate 6 times per day, every 2-3 hours. (Let's start today!)

2   We crawled before we walked. (That makes sense.)

Age 2-5

1   We took changes following our intuition. (Let's get back in touch!)

Age 5-12

1   We ate sweets just because they tasted good. (Let's pay a little more attention!)

2   We did not like when we do to do things like chores, exercise, etc. (Let's make ourselves do these things!)

3   We dreamed, believed, and achieved. (This is what life is about!)

4   We were resilient, forgiving, and honest. (What's so wrong with that?)

5   We were taught not to hang around negative people. (So, why should we now?)

6   We knew that smoking and drinking were bad for us. (So, why wouldn't we now?)

7   We did things that made us happy without expecting a reward. (Think about that one.)

By Doing This, We Find Out Who We Are And Where We've Been.

A.M. Total Being Fitness

Meal Journal

Day 16   Date: _____

Quote of the Day: *You interact with people all the time. When you surround yourself by negative people, you can start to feel negative. You can turn negative experiences into positive ones. For example, if someone takes advantage of you, you need to learn from the experience and from your mistakes. This enables you to grow and become wiser. Becoming angry and resentful will not allow you to move forward.*

Meal 1   Time _____

_____

_____

_____

Water _____

Protein _____

Complex CHO _____

Simple CHO _____

Fat _____

Sodium _____

Meal 2   Time _____

_____

_____

_____

Water _____

Protein _____

Complex CHO _____

Simple CHO _____

Fat _____

Sodium _____

Meal 3   Time _____

_____

_____

_____

Water _____

Protein _____

Complex CHO _____

Simple CHO _____

Fat _____

Sodium _____

creating balance

Meal 4 Time _____   Protein _____

_____   Complex CHO _____

_____   Simple CHO _____

_____   Fat _____

Water _____   Sodium _____

Meal 5 Time _____   Protein _____

_____   Complex CHO _____

_____   Simple CHO _____

_____   Fat _____

Water _____   Sodium _____

Meal 6 Time _____   Protein _____

_____   Complex CHO _____

_____   Simple CHO _____

_____   Fat _____

Water _____   Sodium _____

Total Daily Caloric Intake:

Calories _____

Water _____

_____gms Carb

_____ gms Protein

_____gms Fat

A.M. Total Being Fitness

Exercise Journal

Cardio

Type of Cardio: _____

Duration: _____

Intensity: _____

Calories Burned: _____

Type of Cardio: _____

Duration: _____

Intensity: _____

Calories Burned: _____

Weight Training

Type of Exercise: _____
Reps: _____
Sets: _____
Amount of Weight: _____

Type of Exercise: _____
Reps: _____
Sets: _____
Amount of Weight: _____

Type of Exercise: _____
Reps: _____
Sets: _____
Amount of Weight: _____

Type of Exercise: _____
Reps: _____
Sets: _____
Amount of Weight: _____

Type of Exercise: _____
Reps: _____
Sets: _____
Amount of Weight: _____

creating balance

Self-Assessment Journal

Reflect on the 5 elements of your life. Jot down positive and negative influences and/or experiences of the day. Think about what YOU can do differently to reduce or change the negative and promote more positive. Then put your plan into ACTION!

Spiritual: Did you pray/meditate today? Have you asked for forgiveness for yourself and forgiven others? Have you been grateful and thankful for your blessings? Have you been grateful for the life that has been given to you and do you understand that everything happens for a reason?

Positive

Negative

Plan of Action

Emotional: Did you take a moment to yourself in the morning to pay attention to how you felt, before you started your day? Did you express your emotions instead of suppressing them? Did you acknowledge and allow yourself to feel and experience a range of emotions appropriately, without overreacting? Did you understand the emotions that you felt and not allow them to take you to your past?

Positive

_____
_____
_____

Negative

_____
_____
_____

Plan of Action

_____
_____
_____

Physical: Did you take care of yourself today? Did you eat six small meals? Did you exercise? Did you smoke? Did you drink alcohol? Did you eat fast food?

Positive

_____

_____

_____

Negative

_____

_____

_____

Plan of Action

_____

_____

_____

Social: Who were you around socially? How did it make you feel? Did you limit your exposure to negative surroundings and understand what you felt? Did you give in to negative influences?

Positive

_____
_____
_____

Negative

_____
_____
_____

Plan of Action

_____
_____
_____

Intellectual: Did you plan your day out by writing it down? Did you plan ahead to exercise? Did you prepare your meals and healthy snacks? Did you skip breakfast because you were rushing to work? Did you choose an unhealthy snack because you didn't prepare? Don't forget

Positive
_____
_____
_____

Negative
_____
_____
_____

Plan of Action
_____
_____
_____

A.M. Total Being Fitness

Meal Journal

Day 17   Date: _____

Quote of the Day: *You are affected by what surrounds you. For example, rain and sunshine enable life on Earth to grow. A plant will not grow if it does not get enough water or sunlight. You, too, will not grow if you are surrounded by things that prevent your growth.*

Meal 1   Time _____   Protein _____

_____   Complex CHO _____

_____   Simple CHO _____

_____   Fat _____

Water _____   Sodium _____

Meal 2   Time _____   Protein _____

_____   Complex CHO _____

_____   Simple CHO _____

_____   Fat _____

Water _____   Sodium _____

Meal 3   Time _____   Protein _____

_____   Complex CHO _____

_____   Simple CHO _____

_____   Fat _____

Water _____   Sodium _____

creating balance

Meal 4   Time _____   Protein _____

_____   Complex CHO _____

_____   Simple CHO _____

_____   Fat _____

Water _____   Sodium _____

Meal 5   Time _____   Protein _____

_____   Complex CHO _____

_____   Simple CHO _____

_____   Fat _____

Water _____   Sodium _____

Meal 6   Time _____   Protein _____

_____   Complex CHO _____

_____   Simple CHO _____

_____   Fat _____

Water _____   Sodium _____

Total Daily Caloric Intake:

Calories _____

Water _____

_____ gms Carb

_____ gms Protein

_____ gms Fat

Exercise Journal

Cardio

Type of Cardio: _____

Duration: _____

Intensity: _____

Calories Burned: _____

Type of Cardio: _____

Duration: _____

Intensity: _____

Calories Burned: _____

Weight Training

Type of Exercise: _____

Reps: _____

Sets: _____

Amount of Weight: _____

Type of Exercise: _____

Reps: _____

Sets: _____

Amount of Weight: _____

Type of Exercise: _____

Reps: _____

Sets: _____

Amount of Weight: _____

Type of Exercise: _____

Reps: _____

Sets: _____

Amount of Weight: _____

Type of Exercise: _____

Reps: _____

Sets: _____

Amount of Weight: _____

creating balance

Self-Assessment Journal

Reflect on the 5 elements of your life. Jot down positive and negative influences and/or experiences of the day. Think about what YOU can do differently to reduce or change the negative and promote more positive. Then put your plan into ACTION!

Spiritual: Did you pray/meditate today? Have you asked for forgiveness for yourself and forgiven others? Have you been grateful and thankful for your blessings? Have you been grateful for the life that has been given to you and do you understand that everything happens for a reason?

Positive

_____

_____

_____

Negative

_____

_____

_____

Plan of Action

_____

_____

_____

Emotional: Did you take a moment to yourself in the morning to pay attention to how you felt, before you started your day? Did you express your emotions instead of suppressing them? Did you acknowledge and allow yourself to feel and experience a range of emotions appropriately, without overreacting? Did you understand the emotions that you felt and not allow them to take you to your past?

Positive

_____
_____
_____

Negative

_____
_____
_____

Plan of Action

_____
_____
_____

Physical: Did you take care of yourself today? Did you eat six small meals? Did you exercise? Did you smoke? Did you drink alcohol? Did you eat fast food?

Positive

Negative

Plan of Action

Social: Who were you around socially? How did it make you feel? Did you limit your exposure to negative surroundings and understand what you felt? Did you give in to negative influences?

Positive

_____
_____
_____

Negative

_____
_____
_____

Plan of Action

_____
_____
_____

Intellectual: Did you plan your day out by writing it down? Did you plan ahead to exercise? Did you prepare your meals and healthy snacks? Did you skip breakfast because you were rushing to work? Did you choose an unhealthy snack because you didn't prepare? Don't forget

Positive

Negative

Plan of Action

A.M. Total Being Fitness

Meal Journal

Day 18   Date: _____

Quote of the Day: *Your emotions are "how and what you feel." Expressing laughter or anger allows us to grow just as when we feel pain and cry. Experiencing all emotions is important for personal growth.*

Meal 1   Time _____   Protein _____

_____   Complex CHO _____

_____   Simple CHO _____

_____   Fat _____

Water _____   Sodium _____

Meal 2   Time _____   Protein _____

_____   Complex CHO _____

_____   Simple CHO _____

_____   Fat _____

Water _____   Sodium _____

Meal 3   Time _____   Protein _____

_____   Complex CHO _____

_____   Simple CHO _____

_____   Fat _____

Water _____   Sodium _____

Meal 4   Time _____   Protein _____

_____   Complex CHO _____

_____   Simple CHO _____

_____   Fat _____

Water _____   Sodium _____

Meal 5   Time _____   Protein _____

_____   Complex CHO _____

_____   Simple CHO _____

_____   Fat _____

Water _____   Sodium _____

Meal 6   Time _____   Protein _____

_____   Complex CHO _____

_____   Simple CHO _____

_____   Fat _____

Water _____   Sodium _____

Total Daily Caloric Intake:

Calories _____

Water _____

_____ gms Carb

_____ gms Protein

_____ gms Fat

A.M. Total Being Fitness

Exercise Journal

Cardio

Type of Cardio: _____

Duration: _____

Intensity: _____

Calories Burned: _____

Type of Cardio: _____

Duration: _____

Intensity: _____

Calories Burned: _____

Weight Training

Type of Exercise: _____

Reps: _____

Sets: _____

Amount of Weight: _____

Type of Exercise: _____

Reps: _____

Sets: _____

Amount of Weight: _____

Type of Exercise: _____

Reps: _____

Sets: _____

Amount of Weight: _____

Type of Exercise: _____

Reps: _____

Sets: _____

Amount of Weight: _____

Type of Exercise: _____

Reps: _____

Sets: _____

Amount of Weight: _____

Self-Assessment Journal

Reflect on the 5 elements of your life. Jot down positive and negative influences and/or experiences of the day. Think about what YOU can do differently to reduce or change the negative and promote more positive. Then put your plan into ACTION!

Spiritual: Did you pray/meditate today? Have you asked for forgiveness for yourself and forgiven others? Have you been grateful and thankful for your blessings? Have you been grateful for the life that has been given to you and do you understand that everything happens for a reason?

Positive

Negative

Plan of Action

Emotional: Did you take a moment to yourself in the morning to pay attention to how you felt, before you started your day? Did you express your emotions instead of suppressing them? Did you acknowledge and allow yourself to feel and experience a range of emotions appropriately, without overreacting? Did you understand the emotions that you felt and not allow them to take you to your past?

Positive

_____
_____
_____

Negative

_____
_____
_____

Plan of Action

_____
_____
_____

Physical: Did you take care of yourself today? Did you eat six small meals? Did you exercise? Did you smoke? Did you drink alcohol? Did you eat fast food?

Positive

Negative

Plan of Action

Social: Who were you around socially? How did it make you feel? Did you limit your exposure to negative surroundings and understand what you felt? Did you give in to negative influences?

Positive

_____
_____
_____

Negative

_____
_____
_____

Plan of Action

_____
_____
_____

Intellectual: Did you plan your day out by writing it down? Did you plan ahead to exercise? Did you prepare your meals and healthy snacks? Did you skip breakfast because you were rushing to work? Did you choose an unhealthy snack because you didn't prepare? Don't forget

Positive

_____
_____
_____

Negative

_____
_____
_____

Plan of Action

_____
_____
_____

A.M. Total Being Fitness

Meal Journal

Day 19   Date: _____

Quote of the Day: *Your physical capability is what your body is able to do. When you train you overload your cardiovascular and respiratory systems. This increases your ability to take in more oxygen which is necessary for your body to function When you lift weights, you overload your muscles and increase your strength. Alas: "No pain, no gain."*

Meal 1   Time _____

_____

_____

_____

Water _____

Protein _____

Complex CHO _____

Simple CHO _____

Fat _____

Sodium _____

Meal 2   Time _____

_____

_____

_____

Water _____

Protein _____

Complex CHO _____

Simple CHO _____

Fat _____

Sodium _____

Meal 3   Time _____

_____

_____

_____

Water _____

Protein _____

Complex CHO _____

Simple CHO _____

Fat _____

Sodium _____

Meal 4   Time _____   Protein _____

_____   Complex CHO _____

_____   Simple CHO _____

_____   Fat _____

Water _____   Sodium _____

Meal 5   Time _____   Protein _____

_____   Complex CHO _____

_____   Simple CHO _____

_____   Fat _____

Water _____   Sodium _____

Meal 6   Time _____   Protein _____

_____   Complex CHO _____

_____   Simple CHO _____

_____   Fat _____

Water _____   Sodium _____

Total Daily Caloric Intake:

Calories _____

Water _____

_____ gms Carb

_____ gms Protein

_____ gms Fat

A.M. Total Being Fitness

Exercise Journal

Cardio

Type of Cardio: _____

Duration: _____

Intensity: _____

Calories Burned: _____

Type of Cardio: _____

Duration: _____

Intensity: _____

Calories Burned: _____

Weight Training

Type of Exercise: _____

Reps: _____

Sets: _____

Amount of Weight: _____

Type of Exercise: _____

Reps: _____

Sets: _____

Amount of Weight: _____

Type of Exercise: _____

Reps: _____

Sets: _____

Amount of Weight: _____

Type of Exercise: _____

Reps: _____

Sets: _____

Amount of Weight: _____

Type of Exercise: _____

Reps: _____

Sets: _____

Amount of Weight: _____

creating balance

Self-Assessment Journal

Reflect on the 5 elements of your life. Jot down positive and negative influences and/or experiences of the day. Think about what YOU can do differently to reduce or change the negative and promote more positive. Then put your plan into ACTION!

Spiritual: Did you pray/meditate today? Have you asked for forgiveness for yourself and forgiven others? Have you been grateful and thankful for your blessings? Have you been grateful for the life that has been given to you and do you understand that everything happens for a reason?

Positive

_____

_____

_____

Negative

_____

_____

_____

Plan of Action

_____

_____

_____

Emotional: Did you take a moment to yourself in the morning to pay attention to how you felt, before you started your day? Did you express your emotions instead of suppressing them? Did you acknowledge and allow yourself to feel and experience a range of emotions appropriately, without overreacting? Did you understand the emotions that you felt and not allow them to take you to your past?

Positive

___

___

___

Negative

___

___

___

Plan of Action

___

___

___

Physical: Did you take care of yourself today? Did you eat six small meals? Did you exercise? Did you smoke? Did you drink alcohol? Did you eat fast food?

Positive

_____
_____
_____

Negative

_____
_____
_____

Plan of Action

_____
_____
_____

Social: Who were you around socially? How did it make you feel? Did you limit your exposure to negative surroundings and understand what you felt? Did you give in to negative influences?

Positive

_____
_____
_____

Negative

_____
_____
_____

Plan of Action

_____
_____
_____

Intellectual: Did you plan your day out by writing it down? Did you plan ahead to exercise? Did you prepare your meals and healthy snacks? Did you skip breakfast because you were rushing to work? Did you choose an unhealthy snack because you didn't prepare? Don't forget

Positive

_____

_____

_____

Negative

_____

_____

_____

Plan of Action

_____

_____

_____

What is Physical Fitness?

Physical fitness is emotional, biological, physiological, and spiritual.

Flexibility can and will relieve stress and give you time to think quality, alone to stay centered and better range of motion and help prevent injury. *First, hardest to gain, easiest to keep, the key here is patience.*

Cardio creates more blood circulation, endorphins through the body give you a biochemical high, more energy, clear thinking, almost a sense of elevating your body so you can release and deal with stress. *Second, hardest to gain, easiest to lose, Energy*

Weight Training gives you a sense of strength and power, making you stronger and feel stronger. *Easiest to gain, and hardest to lose.*

Body Composition gives you control over what you chose to put in your body and it is probably the most important because it is what makes you and helps you to live. *Hardest to gain, and easiest to keep.*

Your emotions must be minded as your feelings and intuition stimulate and carry you through your physical actions. Care for your body, your vehicle, as you would care for your car

Stay on Spirit! Stay on the right path in your spirit, as it the force that drives you to move.

creating balance

Meal Journal

Day 20   Date: _____

Quote of the Day: *Your intellectual side what you know. The more you read, the more knowledge you gain. If you are able to apply what you learn and not just "know" it, you are even further ahead.*

Meal 1   Time _____

_____

_____

_____

Water _____

Protein _____

Complex CHO _____

Simple CHO _____

Fat _____

Sodium _____

Meal 2   Time _____

_____

_____

_____

Water _____

Protein _____

Complex CHO _____

Simple CHO _____

Fat _____

Sodium _____

Meal 3   Time _____

_____

_____

_____

Water _____

Protein _____

Complex CHO _____

Simple CHO _____

Fat _____

Sodium _____

A.M. Total Being Fitness

Meal 4 Time _____

_____

_____

_____

Water _____

Protein _____

Complex CHO _____

Simple CHO _____

Fat _____

Sodium _____

Meal 5 Time _____

_____

_____

_____

Water _____

Protein _____

Complex CHO _____

Simple CHO _____

Fat _____

Sodium _____

Meal 6 Time _____

_____

_____

_____

Water _____

Protein _____

Complex CHO _____

Simple CHO _____

Fat _____

Sodium _____

Total Daily Caloric Intake:

Calories _____

Water _____

_____ gms Carb

_____ gms Protein

_____ gms Fat

creating balance

Exercise Journal

Cardio

Type of Cardio: _____

Duration: _____

Intensity: _____

Calories Burned: _____

Type of Cardio: _____

Duration: _____

Intensity: _____

Calories Burned: _____

Weight Training

Type of Exercise: _____

Reps: _____

Sets: _____

Amount of Weight: _____

Type of Exercise: _____

Reps: _____

Sets: _____

Amount of Weight: _____

Type of Exercise: _____

Reps: _____

Sets: _____

Amount of Weight: _____

Type of Exercise: _____

Reps: _____

Sets: _____

Amount of Weight: _____

Type of Exercise: _____

Reps: _____

Sets: _____

Amount of Weight: _____

A.M. Total Being Fitness

Self-Assessment Journal

Reflect on the 5 elements of your life. Jot down positive and negative influences and/or experiences of the day. Think about what YOU can do differently to reduce or change the negative and promote more positive. Then put your plan into ACTION!

Spiritual: Did you pray/meditate today? Have you asked for forgiveness for yourself and forgiven others? Have you been grateful and thankful for your blessings? Have you been grateful for the life that has been given to you and do you understand that everything happens for a reason?

Positive

_____

_____

_____

Negative

_____

_____

_____

Plan of Action

_____

_____

_____

Emotional: Did you take a moment to yourself in the morning to pay attention to how you felt, before you started your day? Did you express your emotions instead of suppressing them? Did you acknowledge and allow yourself to feel and experience a range of emotions appropriately, without overreacting? Did you understand the emotions that you felt and not allow them to take you to your past?

Positive

Negative

Plan of Action

Physical: Did you take care of yourself today? Did you eat six small meals? Did you exercise? Did you smoke? Did you drink alcohol? Did you eat fast food?

Positive

_____
_____
_____

Negative

_____
_____
_____

Plan of Action

_____
_____
_____

Social: Who were you around socially? How did it make you feel? Did you limit your exposure to negative surroundings and understand what you felt? Did you give in to negative influences?

Positive

Negative

Plan of Action

Intellectual: Did you plan your day out by writing it down? Did you plan ahead to exercise? Did you prepare your meals and healthy snacks? Did you skip breakfast because you were rushing to work? Did you choose an unhealthy snack because you didn't prepare? Don't forget

Positive

_____
_____
_____

Negative

_____
_____
_____

Plan of Action

_____
_____
_____

creating balance

Meal Journal

Day 21   Date: _____

Quote of the Day: *Your spiritual self is often described as a belief in a higher being or your faith. You can strengthen your spirituality through practicing your religion, prayer, or meditation. If you are open-minded, your spirituality can be enhanced through life's experiences. For example, when you share in the miracle and joy of the birth of a baby or grieve and reflect on the life of someone who dies, you can experience spiritual growth.*

Meal 1   Time _____

_____

_____

_____

Water _____

Protein _____

Complex CHO _____

Simple CHO _____

Fat _____

Sodium _____

Meal 2   Time _____

_____

_____

_____

Water _____

Protein _____

Complex CHO _____

Simple CHO _____

Fat _____

Sodium _____

Meal 3   Time _____

_____

_____

_____

Water _____

Protein _____

Complex CHO _____

Simple CHO _____

Fat _____

Sodium _____

Meal 4 Time _____   Protein _____

_____   Complex CHO _____

_____   Simple CHO _____

_____   Fat _____

Water _____   Sodium _____

Meal 5 Time _____   Protein _____

_____   Complex CHO _____

_____   Simple CHO _____

_____   Fat _____

Water _____   Sodium _____

Meal 6 Time _____   Protein _____

_____   Complex CHO _____

_____   Simple CHO _____

_____   Fat _____

Water _____   Sodium _____

Total Daily Caloric Intake:

Calories _____

Water _____

_____ gms Carb

_____ gms Protein

_____ gms Fat

creating balance

Exercise Journal

Cardio

Type of Cardio: _____

Duration: _____

Intensity: _____

Calories Burned: _____

Type of Cardio: _____

Duration: _____

Intensity: _____

Calories Burned: _____

Weight Training

Type of Exercise: _____

Reps: _____

Sets: _____

Amount of Weight: _____

Type of Exercise: _____

Reps: _____

Sets: _____

Amount of Weight: _____

Type of Exercise: _____

Reps: _____

Sets: _____

Amount of Weight: _____

Type of Exercise: _____

Reps: _____

Sets: _____

Amount of Weight: _____

Type of Exercise: _____

Reps: _____

Sets: _____

Amount of Weight: _____

Self-Assessment Journal

Reflect on the 5 elements of your life. Jot down positive and negative influences and/or experiences of the day. Think about what YOU can do differently to reduce or change the negative and promote more positive. Then put your plan into ACTION!

Spiritual: Did you pray/meditate today? Have you asked for forgiveness for yourself and forgiven others? Have you been grateful and thankful for your blessings? Have you been grateful for the life that has been given to you and do you understand that everything happens for a reason?

Positive

_____

_____

_____

Negative

_____

_____

_____

Plan of Action

_____

_____

_____

Emotional: Did you take a moment to yourself in the morning to pay attention to how you felt, before you started your day? Did you express your emotions instead of suppressing them? Did you acknowledge and allow yourself to feel and experience a range of emotions appropriately, without overreacting? Did you understand the emotions that you felt and not allow them to take you to your past?

Positive

___

___

___

Negative

___

___

___

Plan of Action

___

___

___

A.M. Total Being Fitness

Physical: Did you take care of yourself today? Did you eat six small meals? Did you exercise? Did you smoke? Did you drink alcohol? Did you eat fast food?

Positive

_____
_____
_____

Negative

_____
_____
_____

Plan of Action

_____
_____
_____

Social: Who were you around socially? How did it make you feel? Did you limit your exposure to negative surroundings and understand what you felt? Did you give in to negative influences?

Positive

___

___

___

Negative

___

___

___

Plan of Action

___

___

___

Intellectual: Did you plan your day out by writing it down? Did you plan ahead to exercise? Did you prepare your meals and healthy snacks? Did you skip breakfast because you were rushing to work? Did you choose an unhealthy snack because you didn't prepare? Don't forget

Positive

_____

_____

_____

Negative

_____

_____

_____

Plan of Action

_____

_____

_____

creating balance

Meal Journal

Day 22   Date: _____

Quote of the Day: *When you were a kid… When you did something good, you were rewarded with sugar, food, or material things. When you were bad, you were physically, emotionally, or verbally scolded. When you were bored, you were given entertainment of some sort. When another kid got something, you had to have it. 85 to 90 percent of adults have issues with food, sweets, drugs, prescription drugs, alcohol, social events, or health problems. We spend most of our money on some form of entertainment. If a car or clothes are popular, then we must go out and buy them. Life is meant to be lived and we are meant to be happy. That is what it is about! Re-think your life and empower yourself to change!*

Meal 1   Time _____

_____

_____

_____

Water _____

Protein _____

Complex CHO _____

Simple CHO _____

Fat _____

Sodium _____

Meal 2   Time _____

_____

_____

_____

Water _____

Protein _____

Complex CHO _____

Simple CHO _____

Fat _____

Sodium _____

Meal 3   Time _____

_____

_____

_____

Water _____

Protein _____

Complex CHO _____

Simple CHO _____

Fat _____

Sodium _____

Meal 4　　Time _____

_____

_____

_____

Water _____

Protein _____

Complex CHO _____

Simple CHO _____

Fat _____

Sodium _____

Meal 5　　Time _____

_____

_____

_____

Water _____

Protein _____

Complex CHO _____

Simple CHO _____

Fat _____

Sodium _____

Meal 6　　Time _____

_____

_____

_____

Water _____

Protein _____

Complex CHO _____

Simple CHO _____

Fat _____

Sodium _____

Total Daily Caloric Intake:

Calories _____

Water _____

_____ gms Carb

_____ gms Protein

_____ gms Fat

creating balance

Exercise Journal

Cardio

Type of Cardio: _____

Duration: _____

Intensity: _____

Calories Burned: _____

Type of Cardio: _____

Duration: _____

Intensity: _____

Calories Burned: _____

Weight Training

Type of Exercise: _____

Reps: _____

Sets: _____

Amount of Weight: _____

Type of Exercise: _____

Reps: _____

Sets: _____

Amount of Weight: _____

Type of Exercise: _____

Reps: _____

Sets: _____

Amount of Weight: _____

Type of Exercise: _____

Reps: _____

Sets: _____

Amount of Weight: _____

Type of Exercise: _____

Reps: _____

Sets: _____

Amount of Weight: _____

A.M. Total Being Fitness

Self-Assessment Journal

Reflect on the 5 elements of your life. Jot down positive and negative influences and/or experiences of the day. Think about what YOU can do differently to reduce or change the negative and promote more positive. Then put your plan into ACTION!

Spiritual: Did you pray/meditate today? Have you asked for forgiveness for yourself and forgiven others? Have you been grateful and thankful for your blessings? Have you been grateful for the life that has been given to you and do you understand that everything happens for a reason?

Positive

_____
_____
_____

Negative

_____
_____
_____

Plan of Action

_____
_____
_____

Emotional: Did you take a moment to yourself in the morning to pay attention to how you felt, before you started your day? Did you express your emotions instead of suppressing them? Did you acknowledge and allow yourself to feel and experience a range of emotions appropriately, without overreacting? Did you understand the emotions that you felt and not allow them to take you to your past?

Positive

_____
_____
_____

Negative

_____
_____
_____

Plan of Action

_____
_____
_____

Physical: Did you take care of yourself today? Did you eat six small meals? Did you exercise? Did you smoke? Did you drink alcohol? Did you eat fast food?

Positive

___

___

___

Negative

___

___

___

Plan of Action

___

___

___

Social: Who were you around socially? How did it make you feel? Did you limit your exposure to negative surroundings and understand what you felt? Did you give in to negative influences?

Positive

___
___
___

Negative

___
___
___

Plan of Action

___
___
___

Intellectual: Did you plan your day out by writing it down? Did you plan ahead to exercise? Did you prepare your meals and healthy snacks? Did you skip breakfast because you were rushing to work? Did you choose an unhealthy snack because you didn't prepare? Don't forget

Positive

_____
_____
_____

Negative

_____
_____
_____

Plan of Action

_____
_____
_____

creating balance

Meal Journal

Day 23   Date: _____

Quote of the Day: *When we look good and we have people around us who are telling us we look good, we tend to have a higher self-esteem, but that is temporary because it is on the outside. When we feel good and look good from the inside, we are truly happy because that is internal and eternal!*

Meal 1   Time _____

_____

_____

_____

Water _____

Protein _____

Complex CHO _____

Simple CHO _____

Fat _____

Sodium _____

Meal 2   Time _____

_____

_____

_____

Water _____

Protein _____

Complex CHO _____

Simple CHO _____

Fat _____

Sodium _____

Meal 3   Time _____

_____

_____

_____

Water _____

Protein _____

Complex CHO _____

Simple CHO _____

Fat _____

Sodium _____

A.M. Total Being Fitness

Meal 4   Time _____   Protein _____

_____   Complex CHO _____

_____   Simple CHO _____

_____   Fat _____

Water _____   Sodium _____

Meal 5   Time _____   Protein _____

_____   Complex CHO _____

_____   Simple CHO _____

_____   Fat _____

Water _____   Sodium _____

Meal 6   Time _____   Protein _____

_____   Complex CHO _____

_____   Simple CHO _____

_____   Fat _____

Water _____   Sodium _____

Total Daily Caloric Intake:

Calories _____

Water _____

_____gms Carb

_____ gms Protein

_____gms Fat

creating balance

Exercise Journal

Cardio

Type of Cardio: _____

Duration: _____

Intensity: _____

Calories Burned: _____

Type of Cardio: _____

Duration: _____

Intensity: _____

Calories Burned: _____

Weight Training

Type of Exercise: _____

Reps: _____

Sets: _____

Amount of Weight: _____

Type of Exercise: _____

Reps: _____

Sets: _____

Amount of Weight: _____

Type of Exercise: _____

Reps: _____

Sets: _____

Amount of Weight: _____

Type of Exercise: _____

Reps: _____

Sets: _____

Amount of Weight: _____

Type of Exercise: _____

Reps: _____

Sets: _____

Amount of Weight: _____

A.M. Total Being Fitness

Self-Assessment Journal

Reflect on the 5 elements of your life. Jot down positive and negative influences and/or experiences of the day. Think about what YOU can do differently to reduce or change the negative and promote more positive. Then put your plan into ACTION!

Spiritual: Did you pray/meditate today? Have you asked for forgiveness for yourself and forgiven others? Have you been grateful and thankful for your blessings? Have you been grateful for the life that has been given to you and do you understand that everything happens for a reason?

Positive

_____
_____
_____

Negative

_____
_____
_____

Plan of Action

_____
_____
_____

Emotional: Did you take a moment to yourself in the morning to pay attention to how you felt, before you started your day? Did you express your emotions instead of suppressing them? Did you acknowledge and allow yourself to feel and experience a range of emotions appropriately, without overreacting? Did you understand the emotions that you felt and not allow them to take you to your past?

Positive

_____
_____
_____

Negative

_____
_____
_____

Plan of Action

_____
_____
_____

A.M. Total Being Fitness

Physical: Did you take care of yourself today? Did you eat six small meals? Did you exercise? Did you smoke? Did you drink alcohol? Did you eat fast food?

Positive

_____
_____
_____

Negative

_____
_____
_____

Plan of Action

_____
_____
_____

Social: Who were you around socially? How did it make you feel? Did you limit your exposure to negative surroundings and understand what you felt? Did you give in to negative influences?

Positive

_____
_____
_____

Negative

_____
_____
_____

Plan of Action

_____
_____
_____

Intellectual: Did you plan your day out by writing it down? Did you plan ahead to exercise? Did you prepare your meals and healthy snacks? Did you skip breakfast because you were rushing to work? Did you choose an unhealthy snack because you didn't prepare? Don't forget

Positive

_____

_____

_____

Negative

_____

_____

_____

Plan of Action

_____

_____

_____

creating balance

Meal Journal

Day 24   Date: _____

Quote of the Day: *Remember that too much focus on any of the following is a negative way to cope with problems: alcohol; blaming others; clothes/external appearance; drugs – street and prescription; entertainment; excuses; food; greed; lies; lust; money; toys/worldly possessions; work.*

Meal 1   Time _____

_____

_____

_____

Water _____

Protein _____

Complex CHO _____

Simple CHO _____

Fat _____

Sodium _____

Meal 2   Time _____

_____

_____

_____

Water _____

Protein _____

Complex CHO _____

Simple CHO _____

Fat _____

Sodium _____

Meal 3   Time _____

_____

_____

_____

Water _____

Protein _____

Complex CHO _____

Simple CHO _____

Fat _____

Sodium _____

Meal 4   Time _____

_____

_____

_____

Water _____

Protein _____

Complex CHO _____

Simple CHO _____

Fat _____

Sodium _____

Meal 5   Time _____

_____

_____

_____

Water _____

Protein _____

Complex CHO _____

Simple CHO _____

Fat _____

Sodium _____

Meal 6   Time _____

_____

_____

_____

Water _____

Protein _____

Complex CHO _____

Simple CHO _____

Fat _____

Sodium _____

Total Daily Caloric Intake:

Calories _____

Water _____

_____ gms Carb

_____ gms Protein

_____ gms Fat

creating balance

Exercise Journal

Cardio

Type of Cardio: _____

Duration: _____

Intensity: _____

Calories Burned: _____

Type of Cardio: _____

Duration: _____

Intensity: _____

Calories Burned: _____

Weight Training

Type of Exercise: _____

Reps: _____

Sets: _____

Amount of Weight: _____

Type of Exercise: _____

Reps: _____

Sets: _____

Amount of Weight: _____

Type of Exercise: _____

Reps: _____

Sets: _____

Amount of Weight: _____

Type of Exercise: _____

Reps: _____

Sets: _____

Amount of Weight: _____

Type of Exercise: _____

Reps: _____

Sets: _____

Amount of Weight: _____

Self-Assessment Journal

Reflect on the 5 elements of your life. Jot down positive and negative influences and/or experiences of the day. Think about what YOU can do differently to reduce or change the negative and promote more positive. Then put your plan into ACTION!

Spiritual: Did you pray/meditate today? Have you asked for forgiveness for yourself and forgiven others? Have you been grateful and thankful for your blessings? Have you been grateful for the life that has been given to you and do you understand that everything happens for a reason?

Positive

_____

_____

_____

Negative

_____

_____

_____

Plan of Action

_____

_____

_____

Emotional: Did you take a moment to yourself in the morning to pay attention to how you felt, before you started your day? Did you express your emotions instead of suppressing them? Did you acknowledge and allow yourself to feel and experience a range of emotions appropriately, without overreacting? Did you understand the emotions that you felt and not allow them to take you to your past?

Positive

Negative

Plan of Action

Physical: Did you take care of yourself today? Did you eat six small meals? Did you exercise? Did you smoke? Did you drink alcohol? Did you eat fast food?

Positive

_____
_____
_____

Negative

_____
_____
_____

Plan of Action

_____
_____
_____

Social: Who were you around socially? How did it make you feel? Did you limit your exposure to negative surroundings and understand what you felt? Did you give in to negative influences?

Positive

_____
_____
_____

Negative

_____
_____
_____

Plan of Action

_____
_____
_____

Intellectual: Did you plan your day out by writing it down? Did you plan ahead to exercise? Did you prepare your meals and healthy snacks? Did you skip breakfast because you were rushing to work? Did you choose an unhealthy snack because you didn't prepare? Don't forget

Positive

_____
_____
_____

Negative

_____
_____
_____

Plan of Action

_____
_____
_____

creating balance

Meal Journal

Day 25   Date: _____

Quote of the Day: *Use your intellectual ability to plan ahead. Plan time for exercise and preparing health meals and snacks. Prepare your meals for a week at a time.*

Meal 1   Time _____

_____

_____

_____

Water _____

Protein _____

Complex CHO _____

Simple CHO _____

Fat _____

Sodium _____

Meal 2   Time _____

_____

_____

_____

Water _____

Protein _____

Complex CHO _____

Simple CHO _____

Fat _____

Sodium _____

Meal 3   Time _____

_____

_____

_____

Water _____

Protein _____

Complex CHO _____

Simple CHO _____

Fat _____

Sodium _____

Meal 4   Time _____   Protein _____

_____   Complex CHO _____

_____   Simple CHO _____

_____   Fat _____

Water _____   Sodium _____

Meal 5   Time _____   Protein _____

_____   Complex CHO _____

_____   Simple CHO _____

_____   Fat _____

Water _____   Sodium _____

Meal 6   Time _____   Protein _____

_____   Complex CHO _____

_____   Simple CHO _____

_____   Fat _____

Water _____   Sodium _____

Total Daily Caloric Intake:

Calories _____

Water _____

_____ gms Carb

_____ gms Protein

_____ gms Fat

creating balance

Exercise Journal

Cardio

Type of Cardio: _____

Duration: _____

Intensity: _____

Calories Burned: _____

Type of Cardio: _____

Duration: _____

Intensity: _____

Calories Burned: _____

Weight Training

Type of Exercise: _____

Reps: _____

Sets: _____

Amount of Weight: _____

Type of Exercise: _____

Reps: _____

Sets: _____

Amount of Weight: _____

Type of Exercise: _____

Reps: _____

Sets: _____

Amount of Weight: _____

Type of Exercise: _____

Reps: _____

Sets: _____

Amount of Weight: _____

Type of Exercise: _____

Reps: _____

Sets: _____

Amount of Weight: _____

Self-Assessment Journal

Reflect on the 5 elements of your life. Jot down positive and negative influences and/or experiences of the day. Think about what YOU can do differently to reduce or change the negative and promote more positive. Then put your plan into ACTION!

Spiritual: Did you pray/meditate today? Have you asked for forgiveness for yourself and forgiven others? Have you been grateful and thankful for your blessings? Have you been grateful for the life that has been given to you and do you understand that everything happens for a reason?

Positive

_____
_____
_____

Negative

_____
_____
_____

Plan of Action

_____
_____
_____

Emotional: Did you take a moment to yourself in the morning to pay attention to how you felt, before you started your day? Did you express your emotions instead of suppressing them? Did you acknowledge and allow yourself to feel and experience a range of emotions appropriately, without overreacting? Did you understand the emotions that you felt and not allow them to take you to your past?

Positive

___

___

___

Negative

___

___

___

Plan of Action

___

___

___

Physical: Did you take care of yourself today? Did you eat six small meals? Did you exercise? Did you smoke? Did you drink alcohol? Did you eat fast food?

Positive

_____
_____
_____

Negative

_____
_____
_____

Plan of Action

_____
_____
_____

Social: Who were you around socially? How did it make you feel? Did you limit your exposure to negative surroundings and understand what you felt? Did you give in to negative influences?

Positive

___

___

___

Negative

___

___

___

Plan of Action

___

___

___

Intellectual: Did you plan your day out by writing it down? Did you plan ahead to exercise? Did you prepare your meals and healthy snacks? Did you skip breakfast because you were rushing to work? Did you choose an unhealthy snack because you didn't prepare? Don't forget

Positive

_____

_____

_____

Negative

_____

_____

_____

Plan of Action

_____

_____

_____

creating balance

Meal Journal

Day 26   Date: _____

Quote of the Day: *If people make you feel bad or uncomfortable continuously, do not hang around them. Be aware of the beliefs of your friends and associates. They can affect you.*

Meal 1   Time _____

_____

_____

_____

Water _____

Protein _____

Complex CHO _____

Simple CHO _____

Fat _____

Sodium _____

Meal 2   Time _____

_____

_____

_____

Water _____

Protein _____

Complex CHO _____

Simple CHO _____

Fat _____

Sodium _____

Meal 3   Time _____

_____

_____

_____

Water _____

Protein _____

Complex CHO _____

Simple CHO _____

Fat _____

Sodium _____

Meal 4 Time _____

_____

_____

_____

Water _____

Protein _____

Complex CHO _____

Simple CHO _____

Fat _____

Sodium _____

Meal 5 Time _____

_____

_____

_____

Water _____

Protein _____

Complex CHO _____

Simple CHO _____

Fat _____

Sodium _____

Meal 6 Time _____

_____

_____

_____

Water _____

Protein _____

Complex CHO _____

Simple CHO _____

Fat _____

Sodium _____

Total Daily Caloric Intake:

Calories _____

Water _____

_____ gms Carb

_____ gms Protein

_____ gms Fat

creating balance

Exercise Journal

Cardio

Type of Cardio: _____

Duration: _____

Intensity: _____

Calories Burned: _____

Type of Cardio: _____

Duration: _____

Intensity: _____

Calories Burned: _____

Weight Training

Type of Exercise: _____
Reps: _____
Sets: _____
Amount of Weight: _____

Type of Exercise: _____
Reps: _____
Sets: _____
Amount of Weight: _____

Type of Exercise: _____
Reps: _____
Sets: _____
Amount of Weight: _____

Type of Exercise: _____
Reps: _____
Sets: _____
Amount of Weight: _____

Type of Exercise: _____
Reps: _____
Sets: _____
Amount of Weight: _____

Self-Assessment Journal

Reflect on the 5 elements of your life. Jot down positive and negative influences and/or experiences of the day. Think about what YOU can do differently to reduce or change the negative and promote more positive. Then put your plan into ACTION!

Spiritual: Did you pray/meditate today? Have you asked for forgiveness for yourself and forgiven others? Have you been grateful and thankful for your blessings? Have you been grateful for the life that has been given to you and do you understand that everything happens for a reason?

Positive

_____

_____

_____

Negative

_____

_____

_____

Plan of Action

_____

_____

_____

Emotional: Did you take a moment to yourself in the morning to pay attention to how you felt, before you started your day? Did you express your emotions instead of suppressing them? Did you acknowledge and allow yourself to feel and experience a range of emotions appropriately, without overreacting? Did you understand the emotions that you felt and not allow them to take you to your past?

Positive

___

___

___

Negative

___

___

___

Plan of Action

___

___

___

Physical: Did you take care of yourself today? Did you eat six small meals? Did you exercise? Did you smoke? Did you drink alcohol? Did you eat fast food?

Positive

_____
_____
_____

Negative

_____
_____
_____

Plan of Action

_____
_____
_____

Social: Who were you around socially? How did it make you feel? Did you limit your exposure to negative surroundings and understand what you felt? Did you give in to negative influences?

Positive

_____
_____
_____

Negative

_____
_____
_____

Plan of Action

_____
_____
_____

Intellectual: Did you plan your day out by writing it down? Did you plan ahead to exercise? Did you prepare your meals and healthy snacks? Did you skip breakfast because you were rushing to work? Did you choose an unhealthy snack because you didn't prepare? Don't forget

Positive

_____
_____
_____

Negative

_____
_____
_____

Plan of Action

_____
_____
_____

creating balance

Meal Journal

Day 27   Date: _____

Quote of the Day: *Accept who you are. Love the things about you that you cannot change. Try to understand them.*

Meal 1   Time _____

_____

_____

_____

Water _____

Protein _____

Complex CHO _____

Simple CHO _____

Fat _____

Sodium _____

Meal 2   Time _____

_____

_____

_____

Water _____

Protein _____

Complex CHO _____

Simple CHO _____

Fat _____

Sodium _____

Meal 3   Time _____

_____

_____

_____

Water _____

Protein _____

Complex CHO _____

Simple CHO _____

Fat _____

Sodium _____

A.M. Total Being Fitness

Meal 4 Time _____ Protein _____

_____ Complex CHO _____

_____ Simple CHO _____

_____ Fat _____

Water _____ Sodium _____

Meal 5 Time _____ Protein _____

_____ Complex CHO _____

_____ Simple CHO _____

_____ Fat _____

Water _____ Sodium _____

Meal 6 Time _____ Protein _____

_____ Complex CHO _____

_____ Simple CHO _____

_____ Fat _____

Water _____ Sodium _____

Total Daily Caloric Intake:

Calories _____

Water _____

_____ gms Carb

_____ gms Protein

_____ gms Fat

creating balance

Exercise Journal

Cardio

Type of Cardio: _____

Duration: _____

Intensity: _____

Calories Burned: _____

Type of Cardio: _____

Duration: _____

Intensity: _____

Calories Burned: _____

Weight Training

Type of Exercise: _____

Reps: _____

Sets: _____

Amount of Weight: _____

Type of Exercise: _____

Reps: _____

Sets: _____

Amount of Weight: _____

Type of Exercise: _____

Reps: _____

Sets: _____

Amount of Weight: _____

Type of Exercise: _____

Reps: _____

Sets: _____

Amount of Weight: _____

Type of Exercise: _____

Reps: _____

Sets: _____

Amount of Weight: _____

Self-Assessment Journal

Reflect on the 5 elements of your life. Jot down positive and negative influences and/or experiences of the day. Think about what YOU can do differently to reduce or change the negative and promote more positive. Then put your plan into ACTION!

Spiritual: Did you pray/meditate today? Have you asked for forgiveness for yourself and forgiven others? Have you been grateful and thankful for your blessings? Have you been grateful for the life that has been given to you and do you understand that everything happens for a reason?

Positive

_____

_____

_____

Negative

_____

_____

_____

Plan of Action

_____

_____

_____

Emotional: Did you take a moment to yourself in the morning to pay attention to how you felt, before you started your day? Did you express your emotions instead of suppressing them? Did you acknowledge and allow yourself to feel and experience a range of emotions appropriately, without overreacting? Did you understand the emotions that you felt and not allow them to take you to your past?

Positive

Negative

Plan of Action

Physical: Did you take care of yourself today? Did you eat six small meals? Did you exercise? Did you smoke? Did you drink alcohol? Did you eat fast food?

Positive

_____
_____
_____

Negative

_____
_____
_____

Plan of Action

_____
_____
_____

Social: Who were you around socially? How did it make you feel? Did you limit your exposure to negative surroundings and understand what you felt? Did you give in to negative influences?

Positive

___

___

___

Negative

___

___

___

Plan of Action

___

___

___

Intellectual: Did you plan your day out by writing it down? Did you plan ahead to exercise? Did you prepare your meals and healthy snacks? Did you skip breakfast because you were rushing to work? Did you choose an unhealthy snack because you didn't prepare? Don't forget

Positive

_____
_____
_____

Negative

_____
_____
_____

Plan of Action

_____
_____
_____

creating balance

Meal Journal

Day 28   Date: _____

Quote of the Day: *Be grateful for the life that has been given to you. Try to understand that everything happens for a reason. Have faith, hope, determination, and willpower.*

Meal 1   Time _____

_____

_____

_____

Water _____

Protein _____

Complex CHO _____

Simple CHO _____

Fat _____

Sodium _____

Meal 2   Time _____

_____

_____

_____

Water _____

Protein _____

Complex CHO _____

Simple CHO _____

Fat _____

Sodium _____

Meal 3   Time _____

_____

_____

_____

Water _____

Protein _____

Complex CHO _____

Simple CHO _____

Fat _____

Sodium _____

A.M. Total Being Fitness

Meal 4   Time _____   Protein _____

_____   Complex CHO _____

_____   Simple CHO _____

_____   Fat _____

Water _____   Sodium _____

Meal 5   Time _____   Protein _____

_____   Complex CHO _____

_____   Simple CHO _____

_____   Fat _____

Water _____   Sodium _____

Meal 6   Time _____   Protein _____

_____   Complex CHO _____

_____   Simple CHO _____

_____   Fat _____

Water _____   Sodium _____

Total Daily Caloric Intake:

Calories _____

Water _____

_____ gms Carb

_____ gms Protein

_____ gms Fat

creating balance

Exercise Journal

Cardio

Type of Cardio: _____

Duration: _____

Intensity: _____

Calories Burned: _____

Type of Cardio: _____

Duration: _____

Intensity: _____

Calories Burned: _____

Weight Training

Type of Exercise: _____

Reps: _____

Sets: _____

Amount of Weight: _____

Type of Exercise: _____

Reps: _____

Sets: _____

Amount of Weight: _____

Type of Exercise: _____

Reps: _____

Sets: _____

Amount of Weight: _____

Type of Exercise: _____

Reps: _____

Sets: _____

Amount of Weight: _____

Type of Exercise: _____

Reps: _____

Sets: _____

Amount of Weight: _____

A.M. Total Being Fitness

Self-Assessment Journal

Reflect on the 5 elements of your life. Jot down positive and negative influences and/or experiences of the day. Think about what YOU can do differently to reduce or change the negative and promote more positive. Then put your plan into ACTION!

Spiritual: Did you pray/meditate today? Have you asked for forgiveness for yourself and forgiven others? Have you been grateful and thankful for your blessings? Have you been grateful for the life that has been given to you and do you understand that everything happens for a reason?

Positive

_____

_____

_____

Negative

_____

_____

_____

Plan of Action

_____

_____

_____

Emotional: Did you take a moment to yourself in the morning to pay attention to how you felt, before you started your day? Did you express your emotions instead of suppressing them? Did you acknowledge and allow yourself to feel and experience a range of emotions appropriately, without overreacting? Did you understand the emotions that you felt and not allow them to take you to your past?

Positive

Negative

Plan of Action

Physical: Did you take care of yourself today? Did you eat six small meals? Did you exercise? Did you smoke? Did you drink alcohol? Did you eat fast food?

Positive

___

___

___

Negative

___

___

___

Plan of Action

___

___

___

Social: Who were you around socially? How did it make you feel? Did you limit your exposure to negative surroundings and understand what you felt? Did you give in to negative influences?

Positive

Negative

Plan of Action

Intellectual: Did you plan your day out by writing it down? Did you plan ahead to exercise? Did you prepare your meals and healthy snacks? Did you skip breakfast because you were rushing to work? Did you choose an unhealthy snack because you didn't prepare? Don't forget

Positive

_____

_____

_____

Negative

_____

_____

_____

Plan of Action

_____

_____

_____

creating balance

Meal Journal

Day 29   Date: _____

Quote of the Day: *Remember, a thought can trigger an emotion. You can change your thoughts to positive ones to change your emotions.*

Meal 1   Time _____

_____

_____

_____

Water _____

Protein _____

Complex CHO _____

Simple CHO _____

Fat _____

Sodium _____

Meal 2   Time _____

_____

_____

_____

Water _____

Protein _____

Complex CHO _____

Simple CHO _____

Fat _____

Sodium _____

Meal 3   Time _____

_____

_____

_____

Water _____

Protein _____

Complex CHO _____

Simple CHO _____

Fat _____

Sodium _____

Meal 4 Time _____   Protein _____

_____   Complex CHO _____

_____   Simple CHO _____

_____   Fat _____

Water _____   Sodium _____

Meal 5 Time _____   Protein _____

_____   Complex CHO _____

_____   Simple CHO _____

_____   Fat _____

Water _____   Sodium _____

Meal 6 Time _____   Protein _____

_____   Complex CHO _____

_____   Simple CHO _____

_____   Fat _____

Water _____   Sodium _____

Total Daily Caloric Intake:

Calories _____

Water _____

_____ gms Carb

_____ gms Protein

_____ gms Fat

creating balance

Exercise Journal

Cardio

Type of Cardio: _____

Duration: _____

Intensity: _____

Calories Burned: _____

Type of Cardio: _____

Duration: _____

Intensity: _____

Calories Burned: _____

Weight Training

Type of Exercise: _____
Reps: _____
Sets: _____
Amount of Weight: _____

Type of Exercise: _____
Reps: _____
Sets: _____
Amount of Weight: _____

Type of Exercise: _____
Reps: _____
Sets: _____
Amount of Weight: _____

Type of Exercise: _____
Reps: _____
Sets: _____
Amount of Weight: _____

Type of Exercise: _____
Reps: _____
Sets: _____
Amount of Weight: _____

Self-Assessment Journal

A.M. Total Being Fitness

Reflect on the 5 elements of your life. Jot down positive and negative influences and/or experiences of the day. Think about what YOU can do differently to reduce or change the negative and promote more positive. Then put your plan into ACTION!

Spiritual: Did you pray/meditate today? Have you asked for forgiveness for yourself and forgiven others? Have you been grateful and thankful for your blessings? Have you been grateful for the life that has been given to you and do you understand that everything happens for a reason?

Positive

_____

_____

_____

Negative

_____

_____

_____

Plan of Action

_____

_____

_____

Emotional: Did you take a moment to yourself in the morning to pay attention to how you felt, before you started your day? Did you express your emotions instead of suppressing them? Did you acknowledge and allow yourself to feel and experience a range of emotions appropriately, without overreacting? Did you understand the emotions that you felt and not allow them to take you to your past?

Positive

___

___

___

Negative

___

___

___

Plan of Action

___

___

___

Physical: Did you take care of yourself today? Did you eat six small meals? Did you exercise? Did you smoke? Did you drink alcohol? Did you eat fast food?

Positive

_____
_____
_____

Negative

_____
_____
_____

Plan of Action

_____
_____
_____

Social: Who were you around socially? How did it make you feel? Did you limit your exposure to negative surroundings and understand what you felt? Did you give in to negative influences?

Positive

Negative

Plan of Action

Intellectual: Did you plan your day out by writing it down? Did you plan ahead to exercise? Did you prepare your meals and healthy snacks? Did you skip breakfast because you were rushing to work? Did you choose an unhealthy snack because you didn't prepare? Don't forget

Positive

_____
_____
_____

Negative

_____
_____
_____

Plan of Action

_____
_____
_____

creating balance

Meal Journal

Day 30   Date: _____

Quote of the Day: *Before you lie down at night and before you get out of bed in the morning, recognize how you feel and understand why… so you may continue with clarity.*

Meal 1   Time _____

_____

_____

_____

Water _____

Protein _____

Complex CHO _____

Simple CHO _____

Fat _____

Sodium _____

Meal 2   Time _____

_____

_____

_____

Water _____

Protein _____

Complex CHO _____

Simple CHO _____

Fat _____

Sodium _____

Meal 3   Time _____

_____

_____

_____

Water _____

Protein _____

Complex CHO _____

Simple CHO _____

Fat _____

Sodium _____

Meal 4   Time _____   Protein _____

_____   Complex CHO _____

_____   Simple CHO _____

_____   Fat _____

Water _____   Sodium _____

Meal 5   Time _____   Protein _____

_____   Complex CHO _____

_____   Simple CHO _____

_____   Fat _____

Water _____   Sodium _____

Meal 6   Time _____   Protein _____

_____   Complex CHO _____

_____   Simple CHO _____

_____   Fat _____

Water _____   Sodium _____

Total Daily Caloric Intake:

Calories _____

Water _____

_____ gms Carb

_____ gms Protein

_____ gms Fat

creating balance

Exercise Journal

Cardio

Type of Cardio: _____

Duration: _____

Intensity: _____

Calories Burned: _____

Type of Cardio: _____

Duration: _____

Intensity: _____

Calories Burned: _____

Weight Training

Type of Exercise: _____

Reps: _____

Sets: _____

Amount of Weight: _____

Type of Exercise: _____

Reps: _____

Sets: _____

Amount of Weight: _____

Type of Exercise: _____

Reps: _____

Sets: _____

Amount of Weight: _____

Type of Exercise: _____

Reps: _____

Sets: _____

Amount of Weight: _____

Type of Exercise: _____

Reps: _____

Sets: _____

Amount of Weight: _____

Self-Assessment Journal

Reflect on the 5 elements of your life. Jot down positive and negative influences and/or experiences of the day. Think about what YOU can do differently to reduce or change the negative and promote more positive. Then put your plan into ACTION!

Spiritual: Did you pray/meditate today? Have you asked for forgiveness for yourself and forgiven others? Have you been grateful and thankful for your blessings? Have you been grateful for the life that has been given to you and do you understand that everything happens for a reason?

Positive

_____

_____

_____

Negative

_____

_____

_____

Plan of Action

_____

_____

_____

Emotional: Did you take a moment to yourself in the morning to pay attention to how you felt, before you started your day? Did you express your emotions instead of suppressing them? Did you acknowledge and allow yourself to feel and experience a range of emotions appropriately, without overreacting? Did you understand the emotions that you felt and not allow them to take you to your past?

Positive

Negative

Plan of Action

Physical: Did you take care of yourself today? Did you eat six small meals? Did you exercise? Did you smoke? Did you drink alcohol? Did you eat fast food?

Positive

_____
_____
_____

Negative

_____
_____
_____

Plan of Action

_____
_____
_____

Social: Who were you around socially? How did it make you feel? Did you limit your exposure to negative surroundings and understand what you felt? Did you give in to negative influences?

Positive

___

___

___

Negative

___

___

___

Plan of Action

___

___

___

Intellectual: Did you plan your day out by writing it down? Did you plan ahead to exercise? Did you prepare your meals and healthy snacks? Did you skip breakfast because you were rushing to work? Did you choose an unhealthy snack because you didn't prepare? Don't forget

Positive

_____

_____

_____

Negative

_____

_____

_____

Plan of Action

_____

_____

_____

creating balance

Meal Journal

Day 31   Date: _____

Quote of the Day: *Realize that you are always going and so are others around you. Allow yourself to express how you feel. Stay true to yourself and others. Always reflect on your days… and plan for your tomorrow!*

Meal 1   Time _____   Protein _____

_____   Complex CHO _____

_____   Simple CHO _____

_____   Fat _____

Water _____   Sodium _____

Meal 2   Time _____   Protein _____

_____   Complex CHO _____

_____   Simple CHO _____

_____   Fat _____

Water _____   Sodium _____

Meal 3   Time _____   Protein _____

_____   Complex CHO _____

_____   Simple CHO _____

_____   Fat _____

Water _____   Sodium _____

Meal 4   Time _____

_____

_____

_____

Water _____

Protein _____

Complex CHO _____

Simple CHO _____

Fat _____

Sodium _____

Meal 5   Time _____

_____

_____

_____

Water _____

Protein _____

Complex CHO _____

Simple CHO _____

Fat _____

Sodium _____

Meal 6   Time _____

_____

_____

_____

Water _____

Protein _____

Complex CHO _____

Simple CHO _____

Fat _____

Sodium _____

Total Daily Caloric Intake:

Calories _____

Water _____

_____ gms Carb

_____ gms Protein

_____ gms Fat

creating balance

Exercise Journal

Cardio

Type of Cardio: _____

Duration: _____

Intensity: _____

Calories Burned: _____

Type of Cardio: _____

Duration: _____

Intensity: _____

Calories Burned: _____

Weight Training

Type of Exercise: _____

Reps: _____

Sets: _____

Amount of Weight: _____

Type of Exercise: _____

Reps: _____

Sets: _____

Amount of Weight: _____

Type of Exercise: _____

Reps: _____

Sets: _____

Amount of Weight: _____

Type of Exercise: _____

Reps: _____

Sets: _____

Amount of Weight: _____

Type of Exercise: _____

Reps: _____

Sets: _____

Amount of Weight: _____

Self-Assessment Journal

Reflect on the 5 elements of your life. Jot down positive and negative influences and/or experiences of the day. Think about what YOU can do differently to reduce or change the negative and promote more positive. Then put your plan into ACTION!

Spiritual: Did you pray/meditate today? Have you asked for forgiveness for yourself and forgiven others? Have you been grateful and thankful for your blessings? Have you been grateful for the life that has been given to you and do you understand that everything happens for a reason?

Positive

_____

_____

_____

Negative

_____

_____

_____

Plan of Action

_____

_____

_____

Emotional: Did you take a moment to yourself in the morning to pay attention to how you felt, before you started your day? Did you express your emotions instead of suppressing them? Did you acknowledge and allow yourself to feel and experience a range of emotions appropriately, without overreacting? Did you understand the emotions that you felt and not allow them to take you to your past?

Positive

_____
_____
_____

Negative

_____
_____
_____

Plan of Action

_____
_____
_____

A.M. Total Being Fitness

Physical: Did you take care of yourself today? Did you eat six small meals? Did you exercise? Did you smoke? Did you drink alcohol? Did you eat fast food?

Positive

_____
_____
_____

Negative

_____
_____
_____

Plan of Action

_____
_____
_____

Social: Who were you around socially? How did it make you feel? Did you limit your exposure to negative surroundings and understand what you felt? Did you give in to negative influences?

Positive

_____

_____

_____

Negative

_____

_____

_____

Plan of Action

_____

_____

_____

Intellectual: Did you plan your day out by writing it down? Did you plan ahead to exercise? Did you prepare your meals and healthy snacks? Did you skip breakfast because you were rushing to work? Did you choose an unhealthy snack because you didn't prepare? Don't forget

Positive

_____
_____
_____

Negative

_____
_____
_____

Plan of Action

_____
_____
_____

creating balance

The Way to Happiness

Keep your heart free from hate, your mind free from worry.
Live simply, expect little and give much.
Fill your life with love.
Scatter sunshine.
Forget self - think of others.
Do as you would be done by.

Try this for a week and you will be surprised.
Raise at your work (great accomplishment)

New house (big investment)

New clothes (refreshing)

Losing 10-20 pounds (self-fulfilling)

Training with Anthony, $65 per session.

Changing your life's direction, outlook and outcome (priceless)

When we look forward to something that makes us happy, we then feel happy.

When we look forward to something that makes us sad, we then feel sad.

If we do not resolve something in our past, when we look back, we will feel the emotion of what we did at that time.

Bottom line:

Understand your past, be aware of your present and look forward to a positive and optimistic future.

The 5 Elements of Life

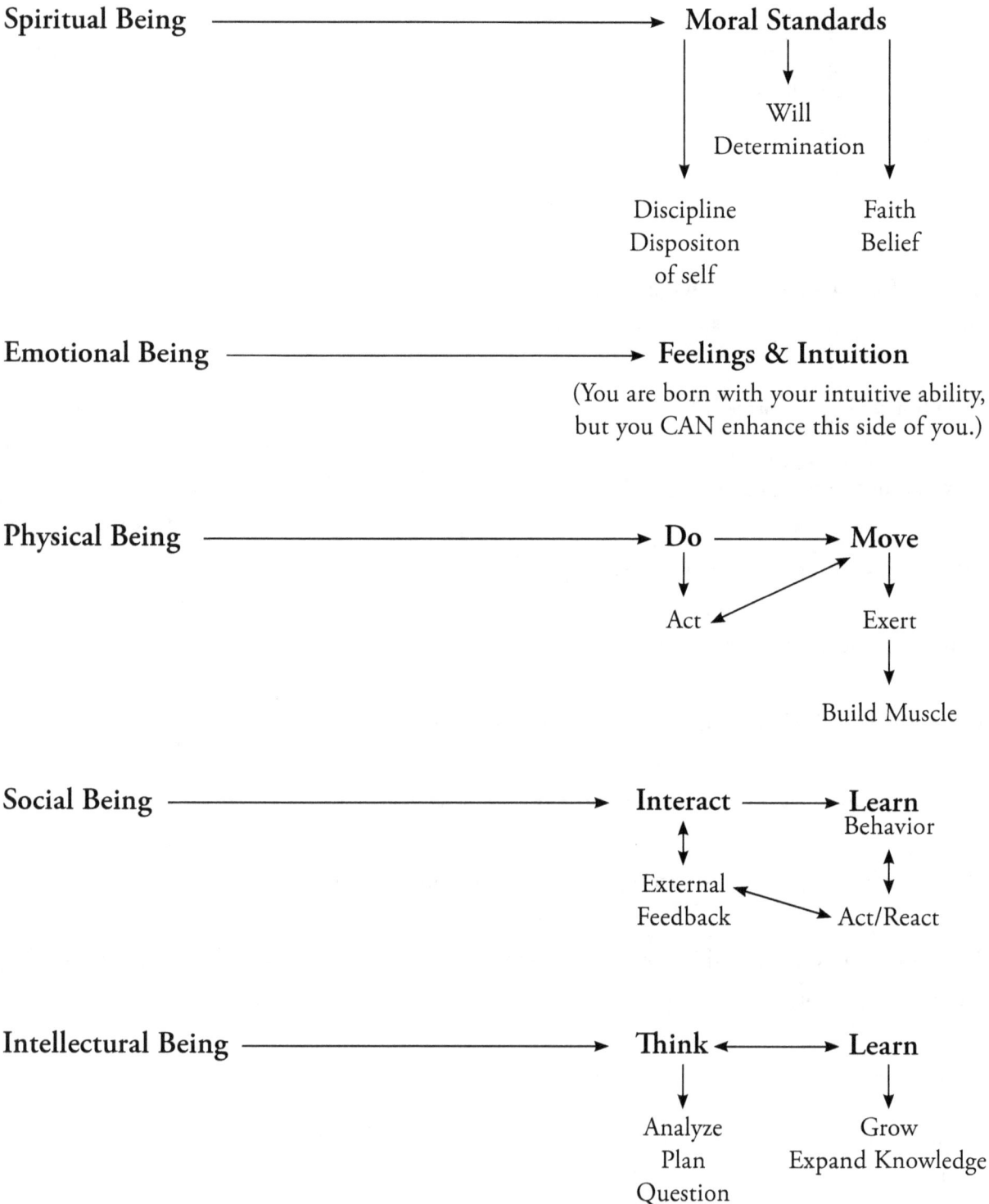

creating balance

Our True Power

Our true power lies inside us and around us.

We can be equipped with the tools needed to positively change our lifestyles and our life choices, diet, and total being through God. God dwells in our hearts when we ask Him and accept Him into our lives. He is also around us and can speak to us through life situations and the people we encounter in our lives. We must allow God to come into our hearts so He can change our hearts (spirit) and give us spiritual life.

The condition of our spirit affects us as emotional, social, intellectual, and physical beings. We are spiritual beings more than we can physical beings. That is what sets us apart from the animals. We are made in God's image. Changing our spiritual condition is the key to making successful, positive changes in *all* areas of our lives:

1. By changing our spiritual bodies, we change our beliefs.
2. By changing our beliefs, we change our emotional actions which changes our physical behavior.
3. By changing our physical behavior, we change our social surroundings.
4. By changing our social surroundings, we change our intellectual thinking.

How can you change your spiritual body?

Changing our spiritual body involves some of the oldest methods in the world, going back to human existence. However, too often, they are taken for granted. They include:

1. Prayer and fasting – Spiritual
2. Expressing and staying in touch with your feelings – Emotional
3. Diet and exercise – Physical
4. Staying away from negative influences – Social
5. Not wanting too much, doubting, or overanalyzing – Intellectual

Now that you have some ideas on how to change your life for the better, how would you like to learn how to experience great emotional, spiritual, and physical blessings in your life? The answer is through fasting.

Why do we get out of shape?
Our physical problems are often a reflection of other problems in our life. In most cases, we do not pay attention to how we *really* feel. Nor do we know how to *deal* with what we feel. Before we know it, it is too late.

How we look on the outside *is* a reflection of how we feel on the inside.

I am *not* just talking about physical beautify on the outside. I am referring to how to carry yourself, your gestures, and you demeanor. These all help other form an impression or opinion about you. Not to say that is right, but we live in society where we are judged unfairly in this way.

For example, how many times have you not slept right, had a disagreement with a loved one that put you in a bad mood, or were preoccupied with something else, only to have someone say, "You looked tired," or asking, "Are you feeling all right today?"

On the other hand, when you are feeling good, having a great day, or have experienced something really positive, you may notice that people tend to treat you a little differently. They are more likely to you compliments and just want to be around you.

We all want to feel good.
When we meet someone with a great personality, what we are really experiencing is their *positive* energy. This energy is generated from deep inside us – from our *spirit*. When we allow our spirit to drive us through life, positive energy *radiates* from us.

Everyone wants to be around people with great energy in hopes that some of it will rub off on us. These people make us feel good. We have all been down at sometime or another. After laughing with a friend or doing something else that we enjoy, we usually feel a little better. These are external influences. If we surround ourselves in positive, then we tend to be more positive. If we surround ourselves by negative, we eventually become negative.

So remember, when we look into the mirror, we are not just seeing our physical shape on the outside, we are seeing what we *are* on the inside. It is important to stay in touch with yourself and how you feel. Don't let others affect you negatively.

The Spirit is the master of the Mind.
The Mind is the master of the Body.
The Body is the master of things that are External.

But...

If you put your socializing and intellect at the top of your priorities in life then,

 Money and things are the master of your Body.

Your body is the master of your Emotions.

You Emotions are the master of your Spirit.

The Spirit and the mind are probably the most powerful gifts that God has given to us.

www.ingramcontent.com/pod-product-compliance
Lightning Source LLC
Chambersburg PA
CBHW081718100526
44591CB00016B/2419